THE JOURNEY

Take the Path to Health and Fitness

Dr. Paul T. Scheatzle, DO, MS, FAAPMR

Order this book online at www.trafford.com
or email orders@trafford.com

Most Trafford titles are also available at major online book retailers.

Printed in the United States of America.

ISBN: 978-1-4269-3364-6 (sc)
ISBN: 978-1-4269-3365-3 (hc)

Library of Congress Control Number: 2010910227

*Our mission is to efficiently provide the world's finest, most comprehensive book publishing
service, enabling every author to experience success. To find out how to publish your book, your
way, and have it available worldwide, visit us online at www.trafford.com*

Trafford rev. 08/06/2010

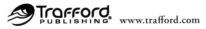 www.trafford.com

North America & international
toll-free: 1 888 232 4444 (USA & Canada)
phone: 250 383 6864 ♦ fax: 812 355 4082

Acknowledgements

To my wife, thank you for all your support and expert editorial input. For my children, thank you for filling my life with joy. To my parents, thank you for always being there for me. To my office staff, thank you for your hard work and assistance in preparing this manuscript. To all of you, I am grateful.

Table of Contents

INTRODUCTION

Begin your journey towards health and fitness. Examine the little things in your life that you can easily change and start today. The journey begins with an examination of different foods and diets and continues with an evaluation of different exercise and rehabilitative philosophies that may be right for you. Along the way, you will learn how you can fit these technologies into your busy life and experience profound changes.

Don't eat anything white seems like such a ridiculous concept that it surely couldn't work. Believe me, if you change nothing else in your diet, do this one thing you will notice real change. This one simple mandate satisfies many of the healthy dietary requirements and it takes much of the planning and lengthy decisions out of the process. Try it next time you go to the store. There are some obvious exceptions but it is a great starting point.

Running may well be the simplest and most ubiquitous form of exercise. Few activities are as accessible, efficient and cost effective. To run, you should wear comfortable clothes, supportive shoes and always look out for your safety. If you are ever injured, multiple rehabilitative techniques and modalities exist to get you back to or even better than your previous level.

Back pain will affect virtually everyone in some point in their life. It is a definite roadblock along the journey to health and fitness. But have no fear. You can overcome it and you will soon resume your quest. Strength training can prevent many injuries by providing a buffer of strength in which you can safely do work. It also aids healing by strengthening tissues while they are healing to ensure that they heal with the proper flexibility and function.

Many different exercise philosophies exist that can be used to maximize your performance and improve your health. Before you start to exercise, evaluate your goals and use them to guide your routine and get medical clearance from a physician. Your physician should support you 100 percent for the simple reason that much of the obesity that is so prevalent in our modern society could be eradicated by these simple diet and exercise philosophies.

Train to improve tone if you want to improve the look and function of your muscles. Based on the path you've chosen in life, adding significant muscle bulk may not be your goal. Other confounding factors such as arthritis in your joints will alter your exercise goals as well. If you suffer from this condition, exercise will provide great benefits.

While traveling the journey to health and fitness, you must learn to fit exercise into your everyday, busy life. If you don't, too many days will pass while you wait for the perfect time to stop and take are of yourself. Learn to balance the external demands placed on your life to avoid detours along your journey. At a personal level, balance your strength, flexibility and diet in your own body. Focus your energy on that which keeps you moving in the right direction and nurture that which gives you positive energy.

10 Benefits of Physical Activity

1. Reduces the risk of heart disease by improving blood circulation throughout the body
2. Keeps weight under control
3. Improves the ability to fall asleep quickly and sleep well
4. Prevents and manages high blood pressure
5. Prevents bone loss
6. Improves blood cholesterol levels
7. Counters anxiety and depression
8. Boosts energy level
9. Helps manage stress
10. Increases muscle strength, improving the ability to do other physical activities

Don't Miss a Beat

Inactive people lose muscle fiber at a rate of 3 to 5 percent every decade after age 30. That's a 15% loss of muscle fiber by age 60!

American Heart Association

It is clear that exercise can treat much of what ails us. Physicians realize this and often prescribe exercise as a prescription. It may consist of certain exercise recommendations, modalities or manual medicine. They do this to allow you to continue to move along the path you've chosen. Ultimately, it's up to you. Choose to move through life with good health, positive energy and with less stress. Begin your journey today!

CHAPTER 1 – DON'T EAT ANYTHING WHITE!

White foods are bad for you. Let's cut to the chase. It is a profound yet simple statement that sounds like an oversimplification, but it is universally true. Processed foods are foods that have had their color and much of their nutrition washed out. Companies do this to allow food to be stored for long periods of time or to alter their taste, but in doing so they lose much of their nutrition. Because of this, the nutrient content of the food we eat is far less than that of our ancestors. If you avoid simple sugar and solid fats, you will eat a healthy diet. The worst types of fat are usually solid at room temperature and guess what? They are white. When faced with food choices, you must always choose the darker item.

Diet trends change and simple carbohydrates have become the most recent culprit. Although created 25 years ago, the Adkins diet has become much more popular in the past 5 years. People use the Adkin's diet to rapidly lose weight. The success of the low carbohydrate diets lies in the fact that insulin causes your body to store fat. Insulin is secreted to help your body digest sugar. The Adkin's diet allows you to eat almost anything except carbohydrates. No longer must you sacrifice the high fat foods that you enjoy. There are several "phases" of this diet. In the induction phase, your body is in a state of relative starvation. You are consuming a high proportion of protein which is designed to trick the hunger mechanism. This occurs because of the fact that you have less circulating insulin with an ultra-low carbohydrate diet. The intent is to use fat for energy. An unfortunate consequence is that you break down some of your protein stores. You will become ketotic and may have the classic "sweet breath" that an uncontrolled diabetic may have. This is not a healthy status to maintain for very long and carbohydrates are reintroduced at a relatively low level in the maintenance phases.

Variety in your diet is needed for healthy living and the lack of consumption of vegetables and fruits has caused critics and most dieticians to discourage following the Adkins diet. In many ways, the South Beach diet is a more balanced approach towards many of Dr. Adkins principles. It follows the low carbohydrate axiom but also is a relatively low fat diet. It stresses the consumption of protein in low fat foods. Limit your fat intake and you'll be healthier and more satisfied because fats are a calorie-dense food. There are 9 calories in each gram of fat versus 4 calories per gram for other foods. Therefore, you will feel fuller on the less calorie-dense but more bulky and substantial foods.

Maintain an ideal weight throughout your life. Frequent dieting creates an unstable environment and makes it more difficult to achieve your ideal "set point". The ideal healthy set point is different for everyone and is largely determined by our genetics. When evaluating diets, realize that they are short-term solutions. They jump start weight loss initially but there must to be a plan for lifelong weight maintenance. Wide swings in body weight are not healthy. One of the major reasons diets fail is because they are viewed negatively and considered to be work. Find a healthy balanced diet that allows you to stay at an ideal body weight and enjoy it! Evaluate what you can have versus what you cannot have and realize the positive effects of this change in your mindset. Deal with the feelings you have about food and how you view passing over things that may be bad for you. Food must be thought of in a healthy context as something we use to nourish our bodies. Appreciate it for its rich tastes and textures and don't use it to fulfill other purposes. Ideal body weight can be maintained with the right balance of enjoyable, high-quality food choices and physical activity. It's the choice you simply must make.

Educate yourself about nutrition and you will make good food choices when you are shopping. Read the labels on the packages and discipline yourself with regards to what you bring into your house. Make a list that includes healthy foods from all the food groups in a close approximation of the recommended daily allowance of each group prior to going shopping. The old saying of "Don't go grocery shopping when you're hungry" is true. It is harder to discipline yourself and make good choices when you are hungry or craving something that will fill you up quickly.

Micromanagement of what you eat is time-consuming and not necessary. Recording every calorie and its classification is a cumbersome process. Because of the rich textures, smells and flavors of healthy foods, preparing and eating healthy can be very enjoyable and you don't want to ruin it by making it feel like work To make it simple, educate yourself where you want to be with regards to fat, carbohydrate and nutrient input. If you make the right choices at the supermarket it will be easy to be in the ballpark. Start with a plan and carry it through from the list you make at home to what you buy at the store. For better or worse, if you bring it home you will most likely eat it.

Don't skip meals when you are attempting to lose weight. This is a habit that is common but not recommended. Breakfast is the most commonly skipped meal but unfortunately, it is the most important meal of the day. What you eat for breakfast sets your "metabolic thermostat" for the day. Ironically, people who skip breakfast are more often overweight. Eat calories spread throughout the day to be most healthy. Steady blood sugars are achieved and consistent energy levels are maintained. It is not a good idea to eat a large meal right before going to bed at night. The calories will be released as you are sleeping when you need them less. You also won't quickly burn the carbohydrates that you consumed because you don't need the fuel to sleep. Your body then will release more insulin to deal with the carbohydrates leading to more fat storage. Furthermore, to aid digestion, it is a good idea to stay upright for a while to let the food pass out of your stomach and avoid reflux. Reflux occurs when stomach acid backs up from the stomach into the esophagus causing the common condition of heartburn.

In Mexico and South America people eat the largest meal of the day at lunch. They eat a large meal then take a rest or even a "siesta", then have a smaller meal later in the evening prior to going to bed for the night. This practice allows them to feel more fully rested and energetic during the day when they are working and gives them adequate waking hours to burn the calories from lunch.

Children must eat a good diet because it sets the stage for their lifelong weight and health. They develop eating and exercise patterns that will stay with them for life and if unhealthy will lead to obesity. Elderly people need good nutrition to maintain their strength and mobility. Protein input is essential to build and maintain muscle at all stages of life, and vitamins and minerals are essential for proper body function. A healthy diet leading to proper weight maintenance will allow you to remain as active as possible late into life. Never is this truer than in middle age, when most of us get concerned about our weight. At this point, people diverge into those who eat right and maintain an ideal weight, and those who do not.

Beyond how we look and feel however, there are many silent benefits to eating correctly. Disease processes are significantly affected by our diet, but they may take many years to develop. Heart disease is greatly affected by diet at all stages of life. Because of the short and long term effects, no matter how old you are, everyone benefits from a healthy diet.

Energy is what most of us crave throughout the day. Energy is what increases your alertness and improves your performances. A steady state level of energy throughout the day allows you to be most efficient and productive. What you reach for to increase your energy, however, is often counterproductive and usually just a temporary solution. A common solution in our society to increase energy is to consume coffee. Unfortunately, drinking coffee just leaves you wanting more coffee. Over time, the caffeine changes chemical levels in your brain so you need to keep drinking it just to feel normal. Without it, you feel listless and sleepy and may even experience headaches. Luckily, as you wean yourself off coffee, this process is reversible. Simple sugars are another thing we reach for when we crave a burst of energy. With the high, however, follows the inevitable crash and you end up feeling tired. The goal is steady energy levels throughout the day to allow us to be efficient, productive, and to feel well.

The right food combinations will achieve the goal of steady state energy and keep blood sugars in an ideal range. Blood sugar control is important for more reasons than previously realized. The importance of good diabetic control has been clearly demonstrated by years of research.

The goal of management is to maintain blood sugars within a normal range. When blood glucose levels are too low, essential physiological functions suffer. A vast array of disease processes result from blood sugars running too high. Insulin is secreted by the pancreas in response to high circulating glucose. With the epidemic of obesity, more attention has been given to insulin's role in storing fat. Obese people have higher levels of circulating insulin and many are pre-diabetic or have diabetes type 2. Diet and exercise alter your metabolism and decrease insulin levels and can prevent diabetes in certain individuals.

Insulin is released in response to ingestion of carbohydrates. Simple carbohydrates consumed alone are the worst because they cause a rapid spike in insulin levels. Even simple carbohydrates consumed with other food groups are better because they blunt the rapid insulin release. A researcher noted long ago that farmers used carbohydrates, i.e. corn, to fatten his pigs, not fatty foods. This revelation led the author to pay more attention to carbohydrates and ways to decrease insulin release by food choices we make.

Seek to achieve balance in your life. Balance with regards to your weight, food intake, and your activity. On a short-term basis, starvation can "trick" your body to allow weight loss, but this is not effective in the long run. Your body will adapt, metabolism will slow, and your weight will stabilize despite decreased intake.

Select situations arise when you want to drop weight quickly. Do this very rarely and never as an overall weight management program. Elite athletes often carry extra weight while training, up to a period close to their performance. They then drop the weight quickly through a variety of measures. This is a dangerous practice that should not apply to the average person.

To lose weight or to maintain a healthy weight, vegetarian diets are a healthy option for many reasons. They require a good knowledge of the nutrient content of what you are eating to ensure that they contain enough protein. Vegetarian diets have far-reaching health benefits including a decrease in inflammation throughout our bodies. Inflammation in our systems has been demonstrated to be an important marker of cardiovascular disease. A test called CRP is commonly ordered now to gauge the amount of inflammation in your blood. Vegetarian diets that are relatively low in fat and simple carbohydrates will lower the measured CRP level. A class of drugs called "statins" has become more popular because of their ability to lower inflammation as well as cholesterol. Much of their benefit however could be achieved through diet and exercise.

Unprocessed, more natural choices will help you achieve an ideal weight and improve your health. Cook your fruits and vegetables less or even eat them raw to preserve their beneficial nutrients and consistency. Nutritionists study the nutrient content of food available now compared to that 200 years ago when we were primarily a farming society. Much of the previous nutrient content has been lost. Vitamin and mineral companies use this fact to try to convince you to buy their products. Although some of this is due to the genetic engineering of our food, much of the loss is attributed to the over-processing of food. Unprocessed foods are more complex with regards to taste, nutrients, and color. Processed sugar and flour lose many of the benefits of the carbohydrate food group and are in effect, empty fillers.

Foods are processed to increase their shelf life. This is more convenient because fresh fruits and vegetables spoil more quickly. Buy fresh fruits and vegetables more frequently because it is much healthier and economical. When you consider cost for nutrient content versus cost per calorie, they are a great value. Sugars packaged in a natural form are consumed with the fiber and nutrients that go with them. They are then digested more slowly, causing less insulin release, and the accompanying fiber provides a myriad of other benefits, including more rapid bowel transit and a slight lowering of cholesterol.

Calories consumed on a daily basis have increased greatly over the past generation. This is due to a large increase in portion size as well as pre-packaged foods. Even though the type of calories consumed and the way they are consumed is important, the total calories remain paramount. Affordability of food in our country has never been greater. Many low-cost, bulk, pre-packaged options exist. The quality of the inexpensive foods however, is not the greatest. Typically they are high in carbohydrates and rich in fats.

Learn the value of food from a nutritional standpoint instead of the most quantity for your money. Weight Watchers has been effective by teaching people to focus on portion size. Each meat item on your plate should be smaller than a deck of cards. Fill the rest of your plate with healthy, low fat, low calorie items. Follow this general rule of thumb with a variety of nutritious foods, and you will have a healthy diet. Portion control cannot be over-emphasized.

Signals which lead you to eat are often not based on a biological need. They arise from a variety of sources including boredom and cravings. To combat cravings, first eliminate simple carbohydrates. This will help you maintain steady blood sugar levels which will decrease cravings. Eating that arises from boredom needs to be replaced with a more healthy behavior pattern. Smart diet choices that you make will eliminate cravings and nurture a great appreciation for nutritious foods. If you eat based on your physiologic needs, over time it will become an engrained pattern that will be easier to repeat. A wide variation in blood sugar means you have poor glycemic control. In a state of poor glycemic control, often what draws you to the refrigerator is not truly a need for more nutrition. If you eat more complex carbohydrates, proteins, and vegetables, your metabolism will remain more consistent and cravings will be eliminated. You can actually eat less and not feel as hungry.

Healthy snacking will lead to weight loss and healthy weight maintenance. In spite of the fact that more calories are being consumed, weight gain does not occur. This occurs in large part to the level blood sugars that are achieved. Snacking also prevents over-eating when you've allowed yourself to get too hungry. The key is to snack correctly. It is okay to treat yourself once in a great while with some sugar-laden sweet, but overall you need to consistently reach for nutritious snacks.

Fresh, raw vegetables make an ideal snack food. Have raw carrots, celery, asparagus or a variety of other refrigerated vegetables on hand and you will always have an easy, delicious snack. They are also nutrient rich, high in fiber, and are not calorie-dense.

In the next chapter I discuss an exercise routine that you can do almost anywhere and at anytime. Best of all, it's free!

Chapter 2 – Running

Fresh air is something we all inherently crave at the end of the day. For those of us who work inside, we miss out on many of the benefits of just being outside. Running provides many health benefits and allows us to breathe some fresh air. Exploring your parks and neighborhoods while running is never boring, and you will see different scenery every time you leave the house. Breathing the fresh air while traveling your parks and neighborhoods can't be beat.

Outside air quality is superior to that of inside air. The unique smells and sounds of the outside add to the experience as well. If you can find time to run during the day, being exposed to sunlight is also a significant benefit. It can help to elevate your mood and stave off the all-too-common seasonal affective disorder prevalent during winter months. Further, sunlight helps synthesize Vitamin D which is important for bone-mineral metabolism.

Aerobic exercise is the primary benefit of running. Because you are using large muscle groups, it is easy to achieve your target heart rate and receive a significant aerobic benefit. The large muscle groups consume a great deal of oxygen doing their work propelling you across the ground. Your heart pumps large volumes of blood at a fast rate to fulfill this need. The speed at which you run is the primary determinant of the heart rate you achieve. Terrain is another factor. Running outside up and down different grades requires more work and utilizes different muscles.

Sustain your target heart rate when running. Because of the consistent effort required, it is one of the most effective forms of exercise in which to do this. The simple act of jogging at a good pace will typically place you in a training heart rate zone and make it easy to achieve this goal. A rule of thumb is that if you are still able to comfortably have a conversation while you are running, you should speed up. It is unique from other forms of exercise such as biking in which it is not as easy to maintain the same level of exertion throughout the exercise session. Unless you stop, you are going to receive a sustained benefit to your cardiovascular and pulmonary systems.

You can reduce stress through running and with exercise in general. Endorphins, which are naturally produced substances in our bodies, significantly contribute to the "runners high." They have a stress relieving effect on our bodies. The runners high is a state of mind that is difficult to describe but easily understood among runners. You feel simultaneously relaxed and energetic. This feeling can be a great motivator. For long distance runners, it can help propel you for long distances. It is as if your body shifts into a higher gear while you are running. The positive effects and a feeling of overall well-being will often linger after you have stopped running.

Isometric exercises can maximize the effectiveness of your running and can be efficiently done while running. This is particularly important if running is the only formal exercise you are doing. To do isometric exercises, maintain the same length of your muscle while contracting against resistance. You will feel your muscle become more firm or it may bulge but there won't be any joint movement. Isometrics can be performed to strengthen a variety of muscles. You can contract your biceps, chest, or neck muscles isometrically while running. This will add significant strength benefits. To do this, simply place your hand against the part of the body that the muscle would move, contract the muscle, and resist the joint movement.

To provide flexibility benefits as well as maximizing calories burned, vary the speed at which you run as well as your running style. You will remain strong, and function within a larger range of motion. If you have a narrow goal such as to run a race as fast as you can, this may not be the best technique. For flexibility, strength, and balance benefits, this is the best practice to mix in with your running regimen. This technique translates to better performance on an athletic field in which different stride lengths and speeds are needed for success.

Posture is an important consideration as well. Good posture is a condition in which we look and function at our best. Good posture while running translates into good posture in multiple positions throughout the day. Pay attention to this early in your training regimen, and it will become an engrained habit. Your postural muscles will strengthen and your spine will align in an ideal position. This will have significant benefits including decreased pain and improved alertness. Good posture while running will further decrease the chance of injury and distribute forces in and ideal way.

Cadence is the speed at which you walk or run. To realize significant benefits, vary your speed while running or walking. Performance on an athletic field requires different speeds of movement. Add bursts of speed or "intervals" to achieve anaerobic and speed benefits. When you train your muscles to work anaerobically, they learn to work fast. Aerobic performance relies on the delivery of oxygen through the blood and is not able to provide the bursts of intense energy. Intervals train your body to use other sources of energy that can improve performance.

Interval training is a quick way to jump start your training program. Short bursts of speed added to an aerobic jog will add speed, strength, and endurance. They force you to do more work, elevate your heart rate, and burn more calories. This is a popular training technique for competitive athletes, but it provides benefits for everyday life as well.

For optimum performance and injury prevention, the construction of the shoes you wear is very important. If you are going to train on a consistent basis, it is worth it to take the time needed to research the shoes you buy. Don't cut cost in this area if you are going to run on a regular basis. Besides the length and width, include the shank, the last, the toe box, the arch, the sole, and the weight (of both you and the shoe) in your evaluation. Have an expert examine your feet and discuss your running habits in order to recommend the construction that is best for you. All shoes will wear out however, and you should replace your shoes approximately every 250 to 300 miles.

Running transfers a great deal of force from your hindfoot to your forefoot. A properly constructed shoe with a soft heel cup, a good medial longitudinal arch, and an adequate toe box with cushioning of the metatarsal heads, transmits these forces in an ideal manner from heel strike to toe-off. This results in maximum running efficiency with the least amount of wear and tear on your body.

For your safety, visibility is important when it comes to running. It is dangerous if a few common-sense measures are ignored. Ideally, cars should always yield to pedestrians. This does not always occur however, so you need to take measures to protect yourself. Run facing oncoming traffic and be prepared to deviate off the road when necessary. When possible, run along secluded roads or in parks to prevent accidents. If you are running at night, wear reflective clothes or battery operated lights that can be attached to your belt or held in your hand.

Besides the risk imposed from traffic, the surface on which you run and other environmental factors provide opportunities for injury. Be smart and assess the terrain, dress appropriately, and always look out for yourself. It makes no sense if the environment is creating risks that outweigh the benefits of your exercise

Variable terrain can provide multiple benefits. The cushioning provided by dirt or grassy surfaces will avoid overuse injuries. The hills and valleys encountered when running outside give you an opportunity to vary your speed and exertion. Running at different angles simply forces you to use muscles differently.

As you get closer to a competitive event, it becomes more important to imitate the same conditions you will face. This is important with regards to running surface as well as the terrain. If you are going to be sprinting on a cinder or rubber surface, begin to train there as well. To maximize effectiveness, do not train in conditions that are significantly easier than those in which you will be asked to perform. Consider instead to exaggerate the difficult aspects of the conditions you will face, and then when the actual performance occurs, it will feel like less work.

Time spent warming up and cooling down is time well spent. It is often neglected by people eager to get into the heart of their workout. Warming up allows increased blood flow to reach the muscles and soft tissues you will be using to exercise. This makes them more flexible and improves their performance. Two of the most important components of warming up are gentle stretching and walking. Walking achieves a gradual warming of your muscles. It is a controlled activity in which you are at little risk of injury. You move your limbs through a familiar range of motion with little strain. Add stretching after you have walked a few minutes to create an ideal routine. Warm muscles, tendons, and ligaments are stretched more easily, and this improves their performance and avoids injury. This is superior to the common practice of aggressively stretching cold muscles.

Join a running group as a way for running to become a social activity. Add this aspect of socialization, and it may become just what is needed to help you stick with your routine. Moderate effort is needed to get an adequate aerobic benefit from running. Your rating on the Borg scale of perceived effort should be 7 to 8. At this level, you should be sustaining an acceptable heart rate elevation. If you are running in a group or with a partner, you will not be able to hold a normal, continuous conversation, but you should be able to communicate intermittently with short sentences.

A running partner can provide motivation and push you to keep going and continue your training program. Subtle and not so subtle competition will creep into your routine and this may inspire you to perform at a level you may not have thought possible. It may be simply not wanting to be the one who decides it's time to stop.

Listen to your body when doing any type of exercise. This is especially true for running. Pain from a specific part of your body is an important cue that signals tissue injury, and is an important trigger to change your behavior. Learn to distinguish this from muscle aching or training discomfort. By quickly assessing the area, you should be able to determine what needs to be changed. It may be that you need to change your routine, take a break or buy new equipment. If you cannot figure it out, ask a professional.

Brace and protect a weak joint by strengthening the surrounding structures. This is particularly true for the muscles around your knees. Strengthen the leg and thigh muscles and it will allow them to absorb more of the pounding that occurs at the knee joints with impact exercises. For your spine, strengthen the surrounding muscles to support the essential framework of your body. This will decrease the forces across your intervertebral discs, protect your back and decrease wear and tear.

It may be that stiffness is causing pain and impacting your performance. In this case, isolate the stiff joint and gently stretch it and the tendons and muscles surrounding it. Be careful to stretch the specific component that is stiff and not the surrounding structures which may already be moving normally or compensating with increased motion. You will be amazed by the effect this simple activity can have on pain relief, performance, and well-being.

Your training goals will, in large part, dictate how far you run. To achieve any aerobic benefit, you will need to run for at least 10 minutes at a time. To achieve a training effect, you will need to run at least 30-45 minutes three to four times a week. Obviously, if you have high level, long distance performance goals, you will need to run much longer.

Add a variety of aerobic activities such as race-walking or biking and you can decrease your running distance, train other muscles, and prevent overuse injuries. If you run less than one time per week, however, you are not going to see a training effect that is specific to running. That is, you may still realize a great aerobic benefit, but your specific running performance will not improve as much. Experience will make it easier for you to judge how far you should run to get a maximum benefit.

Morning is be the best time of day to run for a variety of reasons. People will often ask me what the best time of day is to exercise. The simple answer is "anytime". However, if you start your day with exercise, it will have a high sense of priority in your life and no matter how busy you are, you will have exercised. Running, like eating, first thing in the morning will increase your metabolic rate and energy level. This elevated metabolic rate will last throughout the day and improve your work performance.

Running in the evening has benefits as well. If you have worked all day, you may be more awake, and your muscles won't require as long of a warm-up period. Running will help you relax and burn off the stress of the day and prevent unhealthy stress-related behaviors. It will decrease your desire to reach for an alcoholic drink or over-eat. It interrupts these detrimental habits and replaces them with an ideal alternative.

Running in the middle of the day can re-charge your battery and help prevent the early afternoon sleepiness common after lunch. It will break up your work day and make you more productive and efficient in the afternoon. When you go home in the evening, you will be able to focus your attention on your family. No matter what time of day you choose to run, however, it is a good investment of your time that pays dividends throughout the day.

Fatigue, both mental and physical, can adversely affect your performance. By improving your physical endurance through running, the quality of your work and relationships will improve.

Running will improve your cardio-pulmonary efficiency. By doing so, your body will be able to consume more oxygen and use it more efficiently. Because your brain is an aerobic organ, it will benefit significantly and its function will be improved. Your alertness, memory and attention will all benefit. Further, when others feel physically tired, you will be able to continue. Because of this, running is well worth the time.

Rehabilitation techniques vary greatly. Read on and you will learn what's best for you to get you back in the game.

Chapter 3 - Rehabilitation

Rehabilitation of injuries both large and small is an inevitable part of your exercise routine. To be most successful, base your rehabilitation on your goals and the priorities in your life. Your rehabilitation techniques will differ if you are an injured worker, an elite athlete, or a "weekend warrior". The motivation to return to the playing field will typically be the highest for the high level athlete. They may be willing to do things in the short term that in the long run may be detrimental. For the average person, however, rehabilitation has to be considered in a larger context. Rather than a brief, high-level athletic career, the context is a work career that spans many decades. Because of this, rehabilitation that enables lifelong participation is the goal. Consider what you do for your livelihood when making decisions regarding participation and rehabilitation.

If you are a "weekend warrior," it is important that you are able to go back to work on Monday to earn a living. It is foolish to do activities that place your job at risk. Protect your hands at all times if you need them throughout the day to do your work. Train enough but balance rest versus exercise in order to prevent injuries. If injured, either acutely or through over use, rehabilitation will consist of pain relief, strengthening, and then re-introducing the activities in a safe, pain-free manner.

Muscle atrophy is a concern following an injury because of pain and disuse. Muscles around an injury can quickly lose size, strength, and speed of contraction. Early rehabilitation will prevent much of this disuse atrophy. Determine what type of pain you are having before you decide to begin using a painful area. Is it pain from persistent inflammation of an injured area or is it more aching pain related to the inactivity? An understanding of the healing process dictates when you begin to actively rehabilitate an injury. If you have any doubts, contact a health professional. They will be able to customize a rehabilitation program that will get you back to peak performance as soon as possible.

Begin early gentle mobilization of ligamentous injuries to ensure proper tendon length, strength, and function. This allows for a dynamic healing process. Healing that occurs concomitantly with gentle use shortens the rehabilitation course and improves long term function. For more severe injuries, such as fractures or muscle tears, a longer period of bracing and immobilization is necessary.

If you have good proprioception, you have a good sense of where your body is in space. Restoring proprioception is essential when rehabilitating an injury. Sensory nerve terminals provide proprioceptive feedback and relay information concerning movements and position sense back to the central nervous system. Proprioceptors are present in muscles and tendons and are essential for proper balance. To minimize the loss of this important function, early gentle mobilization is essential.

Joint stability within its range of motion optimizes function and prevents injury. Determine specific areas of weakness or motion restrictions to pinpoint needed stretches or strengthening exercises. An example of this is the shoulder. Scapular stabilizers, which retract, or pull back, and stabilize the shoulder, are the muscles that you need to strengthen prior to strengthening the rotator cuff muscles. Stabilize your shoulder in its ideal position and then you can begin to strengthen the shoulder muscles without further risk of injury or pain. Specific points of weakness along the arc of motion can also be corrected with targeted exercises.

A correct diagnosis has to be made for your rehabilitation plan to be effective. If there is any question, please see a trained medical professional. Further testing may be warranted if the condition is worsening or if any neurological deficits are present. The wrong exercise program will decrease the efficiency of your rehabilitation routine. This is less likely to occur if the correct diagnosis has been made. More seriously, you run the risk of further injury or damage if the wrong program is being performed.

Have your doctor examine you for more serious conditions if any unexplained symptoms are present or if the injury is not resolving within the expected time. This may involve testing to pinpoint the cause of your pain or injury. Tell your doctor if your pain level changes greatly or if symptoms arise in seemingly unrelated parts of your body. He or she will be able to let you know if there is a reason to be concerned.

Isometric exercises, which increase strength when added to an aerobic program, maintain some of the strength around an injured area. Isometric contractions are done by contracting a muscle without changing its length. Because no joint movement occurs, it limits the chance for further injury. Cross training, or doing a variety of different but non-injurious activities, will also help maintain your overall fitness level while you are recovering. The training benefits that you get from doing a different activity will help compensate for the injured area once you resume your normal routine. You lose less strength and endurance than you would if you were sedentary during your recovery.

Maintain your strength and aerobic capacity while you are recovering from a running injury by bicycling or walking. By their nature, they are low-impact and allow healing to occur while maintaining condition. .When you return to running, you will feel rusty at first, but you may discover that you have developed some new muscles that may improve your performance.

It is essential to slowly re-introduce your sport-specific activities when rehabilitating a sports injury. Knowing the right time and the correct intensity are critical for successful rehabilitation. To resume a sports activity, you must first mimic the activity in a safe manner. This serves to re-awaken the muscle memory and the muscle patterns that you used in your performance. For a football player, this may involve running routes or practicing blocking schemes in a non-contact situation. For a baseball player, he would first hit off a tee or do "soft toss" prior to facing live pitching.

Practice is beneficial and improves game performance because of the patterning that occurs in our bodies. This happens in addition to the strengthening and conditioning that occurs. Activity repetition in practice leads to improved patterns of movement. Modify your routine when injured but continue to do what you can in order to decrease the loss in performance.

Inflammation is the body's natural response to a soft tissue injury. Disruption of tissues leads to an increase in circulation and flow of body fluids to the injured area. Stretch injuries to muscles are called strains, and in the case of ligaments, they are called sprains. In both cases, disruption of the soft tissue to some degree has occurred. Inflammation in soft tissue results in warmth and swelling as the body attempts to protect and heal the damaged area.

Ice is the most important modality that you can apply to an injured area. The inflammatory response following an injury is usually more than is needed and can be detrimental both in the short and long run. Ice further can decrease pain and spasticity following an injury, allowing a faster return to more normal function.

Two important goals following an injury are to accelerate healing and to avoid long term damage to your joints. "Cortisone" shots, when used correctly, can help to achieve these goals. "Cortisone" is the general name given to steroidal anti-inflammatory drugs that are sometimes injected into painful joints. They decrease pain and inflammation, help restore normal motion and assist the healing process. They are an adjunctive therapy that allows a quicker return to athletic participation.

Overuse of cortisone however, can lead to weakening of tendons or atrophy of soft tissue. Any one joint of your body should have a maximum of three to four injections per year. Ideally, a cortisone shot is a one time treatment that jump-starts a physical rehabilitation program and makes further injections unnecessary.

Prevent injuries by using correct techniques when training and participating in a competition. How you throw the baseball, block your man, or land from a jump will determine your immediate and long-term success. Work on your mechanics with a coach or trainer. It will have performance and injury-prevention benefits that prevent excessive time spent in the trainers' room.

If injured, take an honest assessment of the injured area and try to determine the cause and prevent future injuries. Was this area weak? If so, strengthen it, as well as the muscles around it. This will improve joint stability and decrease acute, as well as chronic, wear and tear injuries. While strengthening an area, allow enough time to rest and let your body heal. Was this area tight? If this is the case, do gentle stretches to increase your mobility. This will increase the range in which you can safely perform your activity.

Braces, pads and other protective gear can hasten the return to the playing field while you are recovering from an injury. Pads protect an injured area from being injured further by a direct blow. An injured area is at higher risk of further, more serious injury if healing has not been completed. Concussions are a prime example of the devastating effects of another trauma to an injured part of your body. In this case, the athlete should be kept out of competition until all symptoms have resolved. For ligamentous injuries braces stabilize an injured joint and support the tendons and ligaments while they are healing. They further serve as a subconscious reminder for the body to naturally brace and protect the injured area.

To prevent and rehabilitate injuries, evaluate your shoes on a regular basis. Look at the wear pattern. Are you applying force evenly across both shoes? This is the initial determinant of how force is transmitted up through your body. Is the area adequate? Did you match your shoes specifically to the sport you are playing? All of these factors will affect recovery of injured areas from your feet up your spine.

Because of repeated injuries and declining performance, at some point it may be time to quit a specific activity permanently. Knowing when it is time to walk away is difficult for many competitive athletes. Rehabilitating from repeated injuries in combination with age will inevitably cause a gradual decrease in performance. Many competitive or professional athletes choose to go out on top. Others, however, end up being forced out due to the inability to perform at the required level.

Thoughtful amateur athlete will shift their physical activity as they age in order to allow themselves to remain as injury-free and active as possible late into life. It is not worth it to participate in heavy physical contact, such as tackle football, when the goal is to enjoy yourself and stay healthy. People who participate in walking, tennis, or golf can do these activities for the rest of their lives.

The motivation to compete and, for some, to earn a paycheck may cause people to play hurt. Most athletes have a strong desire to return to their activity following an injury and this enthusiasm, in most cases, needs to be tempered. If there is any question, you should consult with your trainer and physician. In many cases, it may be okay to return to the playing field before an injury is 100% healed. In these cases, you need to examine supporting structures as well as your performance and determine if there will be any long term cost to your health.

With proper bracing, recovering areas may be appropriately protected. Masking injured areas with pain medications or injections however, may lead to more damage. Conversely, introducing sports-specific movement to the injured area helps to maintain the "muscle memory" and prevents muscle atrophy while it is healing.

Anti-inflammatories are the most common group of painkiller medications used by athletes. Anti-inflammatories are useful because of the fact that many athletic injuries result in inflammation. When an area becomes inflamed and painful, the body reacts by sending fluid to the region. This process can be detrimental, impede healing and decrease range of motion. Anti-inflammatories decrease inflammation, improve mobility and provide pain relief.

Muscle relaxants, prescribed by physicians, are indicated for short-term use. Used appropriately, they decrease muscle spasm and guarding, minimize pain and allow more motion. Analgesics provide pain relief following an injury and have little anti-inflammatory effect. They range from the milder acetaminophen up to the more potent opioid analgesics.

The primary goal, however, of rehabilitation following an injury has to be healing. Massage, performed in the trainer's room or a therapist's office, helps to achieve this goal and speed the return to the athletic field. Massage can achieve this in a variety of ways. Deep massage perpendicular to muscle fibers can prevent or break up adhesions in ligaments, tendons and muscles. These adhesions can cause a decrease in range of motion and worsen function. Massage further aids healing by reducing edema, improving local circulation, loosening fascia and stretching scars.

Relaxation and pain relief are the most obvious benefits. Relaxing massage is performed by gently applying force along the direction of the muscle fibers. This will increase circulation, create warmth and provide pain relief. It further will aid in removing by-products of exercise such as lactic acid, which can lead to late onset muscle soreness.

Heat and ice remain the most common modalities used to produce beneficial therapeutic effects. When deciding which one to use, it often comes down to which one feels the best. Patients are simply not able to tolerate some modalities. One patient may tell you, "My Mom always used heat," while another will say, "Mine used ice." In general, there are a few guidelines when deciding between heat and ice. Heat and ice can both cause analgesia and decrease muscle spasm. Cold, however, is better for decreasing inflammation and spasticity and for slowing metabolic activity. It is the most appropriate modality for an acutely injured area. Heat is good for increasing collagen extensibility, accelerating metabolic processes and causing hyperemia.

When used as a deep heating agent, ultrasound is known as diathermy. Deep-heating is rehabilitative modality that provides much therapeutic benefit because it penetrates deeper into the tissues. Heating occurs most significantly at the interface of different tissues. It can benefit contractures, tendonitis, pain, and arthritis as well as other pain conditions. Always remember to ask your doctor if you have any questions about your rehabilitation.

Now let's move on to the ubiquitous problem of low back pain.

Chapter 4 – Back Pain

Bed rest was once the primary treatment for back pain. Like using leeches to suck out ill humors, it has gradually become a part of medical history. Absolute bed rest is only indicated if there is an acutely inflamed joint or if there is a suspicion of an unstable fracture or neurological injury. Relative rest with activity modifications is recommended after these more serious conditions are ruled out. This allows healing while preventing the detrimental effects of bed rest.

Bed rest negatively affects virtually every body system. This includes the cardiac, pulmonary, circulatory, gastrointestinal, urinary, dermatologic and psychological systems. Your cardiopulmonary system will quickly lose a degree of its conditioning. Your gastrointestinal tract motility slows, and injuries to your skin and state of mind can occur. With regards to the musculoskeletal system, bed rest will cause muscle atrophy and shortening of tissues. Joints may lose range of motion or develop contractures. Bones may lose calcium and become osteoporotic. Work with your health care professional and make a concerted effort to minimize the harmful effects of bed rest by using your muscles and remaining as active as possible.

Imaging tests may be ordered if there is a suspicion of more serious pathology. X-rays are the most common test done for low back pain after the history and physical are completed. X-rays provide your doctor with a shadow image and most clearly demonstrate any bone problems. These include fractures and degenerative changes. To see soft tissue more clearly, other more advanced testing is needed.

MRI or magnetic resonance imaging gives a clear picture of the soft tissues. This test, however, is quite expensive and should be ordered only when there is a high index of suspicion for serious pathology. Although it is a popular test, ordering it without a specific indication may reveal "abnormal" findings of limited significance and cause further confusion. Most middle-aged people will have some pathology that has little meaning outside the context of a good history and physical examination.

Your doctor may further order a CT or "cat" scan to more clearly look at a cross-section of bony architecture. Myelograms are a test in which dye is injected into your spinal column to look for areas of pinched nerves. Because of the high quality images that MRIs can now provide, myelograms are less commonly ordered. Electromyography or EMG/NCV is a test performed by a Physical Medicine and Rehabilitation specialist or a Neurologist that measures nerve conduction velocities and electrical activity from your muscles. It provides functional information and helps your doctor to put all the information together and make the correct diagnosis.

Physical Therapists are an integral part of the rehabilitation team that treats low back pain. They work with you to provide pain relief, strengthening and education about the care of your back. Most physical therapists have a master's degree and they can be a valuable resource. They may lead "back schools," where people come to learn about the care and treatment of their back. These include education regarding exercise, proper lift techniques as well as good body mechanics.

After evaluating a patient with back pain, I will commonly write a prescription for lumbar spine stabilization as well as postural training. This usually occurs over a period of two to three times per week for one to two months. Following this, patients advance to an independent home exercise program. A program such as this can have short term benefits of strengthening and pain relief and long term ones including injury prevention and a healthier lifestyle.

Osteopathic manipulative therapy is a form of manual medicine that was begun in the late 1800's. It is a form of treatment of back pain that involves using the physician's hands to treat the patient. Other forms of manual therapy include chiropractic medicine, neuromuscular and massage therapy. To be most effective, these need to occur in conjunction with an exercise program.

Ideally, manual medicine is a direct extension of the physical exam. When the doctor or therapist is palpating a painful or dysfunctional part of your back, they can receive a great deal of information about your problem. They can then use this information immediately to treat you in a direct or indirect way. To treat it directly, the professional engages barriers and then gently applies force to restore more normal range of motion. Indirectly, they move away from the barriers and allow natural forces to work to restore balance.

Interventional techniques are something that your doctor may offer if your pain is not going away. They include many injections that are done to treat pain. Epidural injections are indicated primarily for arm or leg pain caused by pinched nerves in your neck or back. They are more effective in treating the effects of the pinched nerve in your arms or legs than in treating your neck or back pain. You may need a facet block if you have more pain in the posterior aspect of your spinal column and if it hurts more with extension or when you lean back. Focal nerve blocks are done in multiple parts of your body and target specific painful areas. The goal is to improve motion and decrease pain long after the medicine has worn off. Nerve blocks are an effective part of a comprehensive pain management program that aims to improve your level of function as well as decrease your pain.

Bowel or bladder incontinence or progressive neurological deficits, such as paralysis, are the two absolute back surgery indications. Back surgery is rarely indicated if back pain is the only symptom and it may be detrimental in the long run. It is more helpful for leg pain resulting from a pinched nerve in your back. Decompression refers to the surgical removal of disc and arthritic material that is pressing on your nerve root. Fusion is performed to stabilize the spine when there is evidence of instability.

Until recently it was felt that if a herniated disc was present, the patient needed back surgery. It has been shown that there are many other ways to treat herniated discs. Forty percent of normal patients age forty to sixty have MRI evidence of bulging or herniated discs. If these were surgically resected, the patient would not benefit. To provide the best care, we treat the patient, not the imaging studies.

The Kirkaldy-Willis degenerative cascade is a model created to describe the short and long term effects of injury to your back. Initially your body will react to the pain by naturally bracing or stabilizing an injured segment. Because of injury and disuse, this area may become lax or hypermobile. This instability will lead to further permanent injury and degenerative changes. These degenerative changes, including bony spurs and thickening of supporting ligaments, are your body's natural reaction to stabilize your spine.

Spine stabilization exercises are an attempt to disrupt this cascade before permanent anatomic changes occur. Think of your back as a tent, with your spine as the center pole. Train all of the muscles around your spine to stabilize and protect it. To do spine stabilizing exercises, strengthen your abdominal muscles in the front and back extensor muscles posteriorly. The proper balance of strength and flexibility front to back and side to side is essential to keep your back healthy.

Depression is a condition of persistent sadness and lack of motivation that all too often is present with chronic back pain. It is not clear which occurs first, but both conditions are intertwined. Back pain has the unfortunate ability to affect all aspects of your life. Anti-depressants, though not treating the pain directly, can be helpful to improve function and are commonly prescribed. Cognitive-behavioral therapy by a psychologist identifies maladaptive thinking processes and teaches valuable coping mechanisms.

A model has been devised that depicts the different aspects of your life as a series of interlocking circles that connect and interact to make us who we are. In this context, it is easy to see the devastating effect low back pain can have when it infiltrates all of these aspects. It intersects with your physical, spiritual and emotional being and changes your life. Most devastating is its ability to shrink these circles and diminish your fullness of life.

Work to improve your quality of life and function by trying to get a good night's sleep. An early marker of improvement in your back pain is restful sleep. Conversely, it is essential to experience restorative sleep in order to decrease pain and feel an increased level of energy and alertness. You will sleep better if you have less pain and you will have less pain if you get a good night's sleep. To do this, you must have good sleep hygiene. This means a consistent bed time, avoidance of caffeine late in the day, decreased noise and distractions, and a mattress that is appropriate for you. To support your spine, this means a mattress that is usually firm or semi-firm.

Schedule enough time in your day to allow your mind and body to rest. Adults require approximately eight hours of sleep per night. In our modern society, this is much more than the average American sleeps. If sleep problems persist despite sleep hygiene changes see your doctor. He or she may recommend a formal sleep evaluation, with an overnight stay at a sleep center, and then provide medications or order further testing.

All athletes need to condition themselves in order to maximize their performance. For the back pain patient this is true as well. An exercise physiologist can be a valuable part of the rehabilitation team that is working towards this goal. The role of the exercise physiologist is to apply physiology to your conditioning program in a holistic way. By doing so, they look at you as a whole person and how all your different systems interact. They focus on multiple different organ systems, such as the cardiopulmonary or neuromuscular systems, in the context of the whole person.

In certain patients, exercise physiologists may create an exercise program that maximizes the athlete's ability to use oxygen. In others, they may need to focus more on strength. In those cases, they would prescribe an anaerobic, resistance regimen. The exercise physiologist is a valuable team member because he understands the structure and function of the organ systems. He helps each athlete to recover from injuries and perform at their highest level.

Personalized exercise instruction may be what is needed to jump start or energize your exercise routine. Working with a personal trainer can optimize your exercise outcomes whether or not you are experiencing back pain. A trainer can challenge you and point you in the right direction. They also should have a great deal of knowledge regarding the equipment where they work so they can make sure you are using it correctly.

Have an evaluation of your strengths and weaknesses performed and list your goals prior to beginning a program directed by a personal trainer. Armed with this information, they can more personally direct you in specific exercises to achieve your goals. They can provide instruction on the use of machines or "spot" you to help avoid injury. They further will direct specific exercises towards areas of weakness. Over time, your need for a personal trainer will diminish as you become more experienced and comfortable with your exercise routine.

Pain in the posterior part of your back that is made worse with extension suggests specific pathology that needs to be treated differently. Spinal stenosis and facet syndrome are two of the most common causes of pain with extension. Flexion exercises are a necessary part of your exercise routine in these cases. A Williams Flexion exercise program involves using muscles that tend to curl you up into a ball. These include exercises using your stomach and hip muscles. This allows injured areas to heal and pain to subside. Once you can extend your back and stand up, comfortably introduce extension and postural exercises to avoid a permanently flexed posture. While doing flexion exercises, the pain and irritation from the posterior elements of your back should recede. Once it does, you can then start stretching and strengthening your back from all angles to achieve good postural balance.

Unfortunately, we live so much of our lives in a flexed position. Picture yourself at work. If you are in an office job, you work in a seated position. Your hips and knees are flexed. Your neck and back are bent forward and your shoulders are drooped. To counteract this, extension exercises are very important. For low back pain, they are essential. By doing extension exercises, you can decompress and distract your low back. A whole physical therapy philosophy called McKenzie exercises is based on extension exercises. They are built on the philosophy of the centralization of pain by extending and distracting the spine. They decrease the amount of pain in the arms or legs and limit the pain to the smallest amount possible in the axial or central spine.

To envision how a disc bulges or herniates when it is compressed, think of the discs in your back as jelly doughnuts. Annular fibers contain the disc material in an anatomic position but when they are disrupted, disc material can protrude out and cause pain. By doing extension exercises you can distract your disc and draw the jelly material back in. When the jelly leaks out, due to injury or degeneration, pressure and inflammation causes pain in your low back. If it abuts a spinal nerve, it may radiate down your leg, a condition commonly known as sciatica.

Body mechanics are important for both injury prevention as well as recovery. Ideal body weight is a key component of the forces placed upon your spine. The benefits of weight loss are great because forces are better transferred through your spine and are not displaced so far anteriorly. In order to achieve good body mechanics, you need to balance the forces of weight, flexibility and strength. Your body composition will play a large part in your ability to achieve this balance.

If you have a large stomach, your center of gravity will be displaced forward. This exponentially increases the amount of force transmitted through your spine. To compensate, you have to increase the sway, or lordosis, in your low back to maintain balance. This is a recipe for low back pain. Further, the increased weight you carry applies more force from all angles as your body moves the extra load. Proper body mechanics means moving and lifting in a balanced, safe way. Increased weight makes this more difficult while at the same time increasing the wear and tear on your low back.

Circulation of nutrients and fluids to the intervertebral discs is essential to maintain their health. Smoking robs the blood of oxygen and delivers toxic substances like carbon monoxide. Further, chemicals in cigarettes vasoconstrict your blood vessels thereby decreasing the total amount of blood that reaches your discs. Because of this, spine surgeons insist that patients quit smoking before undergoing back surgery.

Next to job dissatisfaction, smoking may be the most important predictor of low back pain in the workplace. Because of the chronic lack of fluid, nutrients and oxygenation, the tissue of smokers is simply not as healthy. Other unhealthy lifestyle choices that frequently go along with smoking conspire to make maters worse. Smokers are less likely to exercise and may drink more alcohol which magnifies the detrimental effects.

In the following chapter, I will provide an overview of strength training that you can use to guide your resistance exercise program.

Chapter 5 – Strength Training

Strength is an invaluable asset for any athlete, casual or competitive. Strength gives you the ability to produce more force. Weight training provides multiple benefits that improve performance and prevent injury. Further, weight lifting can give you the confidence to know that you are looking and performing your best.

Weight training will provide improvements in strength from day one. Before you see any size or tone differences you will notice a training effect. Almost immediately, your muscles are responding to the increased demands by learning to produce more force. Because of the distribution of motor centers in the brain, you can even see benefits on the opposite side of your body.

The teenage years are when it is acceptable to begin weight training. Prior to these years, children should not do resistance training. It may place them at too high of a risk for injury and may effect their growth plates and flexibility. For children, emphasize enjoyment of the activity while they acquire valuable physical, social and life skills. The repetitious nature of weight training may cause a youngster to become bored and to lose interest in the activity. Flexibility, balance, coordination and enjoyment of the activity are most important prior to the teen years.

As hormone levels change in puberty, weight training will allow teens to more easily build muscles and increase strength. You will be able to see size and strength results from your work. Tailor your strength regimen to the activity you do the most if you have chosen to try to excel in specific sports. Focus more attention on muscles that will be called on to do more work. Increase your muscle strength and it will help virtually every aspect of your performance and aid in injury prevention.

The epidemic of obesity has extended in recent years to children and teenagers. Because of this, there are thousands of teenagers unable to participate fully in speed-based sports. Weight lifting provides them an outlet in which they can excel. For them, strength training can give them an edge and allow them to contribute to their team. Increased strength will also improve their mobility throughout their life.

With increased mobility, an obese person may be able to improve their overall level of conditioning. This demonstrates how the effects of the weight training can translate to other aspects of your life. Further, the improved strength may increase their self confidence and self esteem and impact their whole life in a positive way.

Falls in the elderly are devastating to the individual as well as society. Less than half of elderly people who fall and break their hip ever regain their previous functional status. Gait and strength training provides benefits that decrease the number of falls. It improves an elderly person's mobility and balance. By being stronger, the injurious effects of falling will also be minimized. Elderly people who remain active will also retain better cognition.

Much of our lifetime loss of strength and mobility is due to a decreased level of activity as opposed to any specific age-related physiological changes that occur. Unless a disease process develops, significant strength losses that occur before your 60's cannot be explained by any natural muscle changes. I tell my patients that if you remain active and do some type of resistance or strength building activity, you should be able to maintain most of your strength throughout your lifetime.

Aerobic benefits are achieved by weight training as well. Weight training typically is thought of as an anaerobic activity. This means that it is less of an oxygen-dependant activity than some endurance activities, like running. There are many ways, however, that weight training crosses over to the aerobic realm. Sustained heart rate elevations can be achieved by performing a high number of repetitions when weight training. As muscle groups grow, peripheral circulation will improve due to the fact that muscle is much more vascular than adipose. You improve your oxygen carrying capacity and ability to remove waste when you have better circulation.

With improved strength, you will also be able to sustain your workout longer. Increased strength will stabilize and protect the weight bearing joints needed for aerobic exercise. Strengthening your legs prevents them from being the factor that causes you to stop your endurance workout. When you strengthen your base of support, the benefits cross over and improve your performance in all your activities.

Controlled movements are essential with weight training. Rapid or uncoordinated movements place you at risk for injury and are less effective. Rapid movements may allow your joint to "coast" through certain parts of the arc of motion. You will not realize any strength benefits at these points. Controlled movements allow you to maintain contraction of your muscles throughout their movement, which protects your joints and muscles. Use the proper form in conjunction with good posture, and you will receive the most benefit.

To breathe correctly while lifting, you should exhale at the point when you are applying the most force. Never hold your breath. A Valsalva maneuver, or forceful exhalation against a closed airway, results in an increase in intrathoracic pressure and interferes with venous return to the heart. Holding your breath or exhaling against a closed airway significantly increases the pressure inside your body and puts you at risk for many different injuries. These could include disk herniation, vascular or soft tissue injuries.

Remember your posture, no matter what muscles you are exercising, and always use proper form. The postures you hold while exercising are the ones you will most likely maintain subconsciously throughout the day. Use the muscles that hold your body in the proper alignment because this will provide a biomechanical advantage. Hold your stomach in and keep your shoulders back when you are doing curls, walking, or any exercise, and you will see greater results.

Free weights isolate specific muscles and provide a significant benefit over other forms of strength training. The need to control the weight in every plane of movement maximizes their effectiveness. Weight machines allow movement only along a predetermined path so you don't receive this added benefit. Free weights are portable and less expensive than resistance machines. For most people, they are the place to start when beginning a strength-training program.

Free weights can be used to strengthen virtually every muscle in the body. They provide maximum benefit because they are not supported by any other means except the constant force of the athlete. To control the weight in multiple planes, different muscles are called upon to act together. Frequently they act in opposing manners to provide smooth stable movements. If you move a free weight through specific arcs of motion while controlling it in all planes you will realize increases in strength and performance. The success of the P90X program demonstrates this principle.

The main value of using exercise machines is the added safety they provide. Weight machines are typically grouped together in gyms in designated areas where people can go to work many of their muscles. If you do the circuit of available machines, chances are, you have worked most of your muscles. They usually provide an adequate variety and a safe workout. Further, they are designed to be simple to use, and you can get started on your exercise routine on the first day.

Resistance training on weight machines however, is less representative of real-life activities than free-weight lifting. Often, the machine does much of the joint stabilization for you, and you simply use the muscles to move your joint through the machine's range of motion. This may be safer but it does not develop proprioception, balance or joint stability as much as resistance training with free weights.

Individuals find motivation to stick to their weight training program in a variety of ways. Often people will wonder if they should work out at home or join a gym. It comes down to the simple fact that you should work out wherever you are most likely to do so. It needs to be convenient and affordable. You may join a gym simply because lifting weights in your basement is too boring. Do whatever it takes to keep yourself motivated. Set new goals. Try a greater variety of exercises. For many people, however, the choice is simply based on cost. Gym memberships can be very expensive. The cost per visit will be astronomical if you go rarely.

For the money, there is no better value than lifting free weights at home. Ultimately however, the best exercise is simply going to be the one you do. Almost any exercise is better than none. Do what it takes to keep yourself going when you feel yourself losing interest. Put a TV in your basement or find an exercise partner. Just do it.

Anabolic steroids, chemicals used to help build muscle, have been part of competitive weight lifting for many years. Only recently have professional and amateur sports organizations stepped up their efforts to rid their groups of steroids. The use of steroids in a healthy athlete is never justified. Most people nowadays consider it to be cheating, because it creates an unfair advantage. Although they may help to build muscle in the short run, long term, they lead to negative side effects on multiple organs of your body.

Our bodies produce steroids in a balanced fashion that maintains our metabolism and allows us to grow. In rare cases when this system fails, such as a cachectic, frail elderly person, or a patient with a metabolic disease, steroids may be needed to regain that balance. A healthy person should not take steroids. They are illegal and unhealthy. A steroid user gambles that the side effects will not significantly outweigh the potential benefits. Consider also the shame and embarrassment that occurs when they are caught cheating, and it is clear that it is simply not worth it.

There is no better motivator than the fact that the benefits of weight training can be felt day one with no significant learning curve. Before you ever notice an increase in size of the muscle you are working, it will perform better. It does not require a great deal of coordination or athletic ability to begin a weight training program. What you will find however, is that the increased strength you quickly obtain will translate to improved performance in many measures. Your speed will be more explosive, your throws longer and your agility improved. You directly strengthen the muscles with weight lifting that are responsible for these activities and indirectly strengthen supporting structures. Strengthening activities will further cross the midline and provide benefits to the same muscles on the opposite sides of your body.

Isometric exercises are performed by contracting a muscle while preventing joint movement. The contraction produces increased tension at a constant overall length. They provide great strength improvements while minimizing the force across a joint. It is a form of exercise that can be done anywhere and one that requires no equipment.

"Slow burns" or slow motion weight training enables you to work your muscles to the point of fatigue to add size and strength. With concentric isokinetic exercises, a contracting muscle shortens at a constant rate of speed. The point of slow motion isokinetic exercises is to lift heavier weights fewer times and at a slower speed. In doing so, you are applying near maximum force while both flexing and extending your joint. Better technique is usually achieved as you are unable to do any "jerking" type movements or make postural changes to lift the weight easier. They isolate and push your muscle to do maximum work throughout the full range of motion.

Concentric contractions shorten a muscle. Eccentric exercises are one sin which you contract your muscle as it is lengthening. "Negatives" or eccentric contractions are an important part of your weight training routine. They enable you to exert maximum force as your muscle is lengthening. As you control the extension of a joint such as your biceps, you will be able to work your muscle to the point of fatigue and near failure.

The agonist/antagonist relationship is important in weight training to stabilize joints, avoid injury and maximize performance. Antagonistic muscles, such as the hamstring muscles coupled with your quadriceps, fire to provide an opposite, balancing force that helps control a movement. They are essential for isotonic exercises in which a contracting muscle shortens against a constant load. Isotonic exercises are ones in which you lift a constant weight at any speed. Done eccentrically, they highlight this relationship and are an essential part of any strength training routine.

By making daily tasks easier, weight training can make you feel more energetic. Do weight training and you will achieve greater strength and increase your energy reserve. A smaller percentage of your total strength is needed for daily activities. Because of this, you will be more efficient and less prone to injury.

By gaining strength, you will be able to do more work while perceiving that you are doing less. You feel more energetic while you are doing a task. You feel more energetic at the end of the day because you may have barely tapped into your potential. If you train with twenty pound dumbbells, when you must lift a ten pound box at work, it will be easy to do. By training with heavy weights, you can develop energy and strength reserves that you can use throughout the day.

Vary the intensity of your workouts on a daily basis to ensure success of a long term program. This is the concept of "periodization". It incorporates periods in which you tear down your muscles and then build them up again. Strenuous exercise is followed by less intense work or complete rest. Allow the needed time for recovery to achieve the appropriate balance.

Competitive athletes will use the concept of periodization as they approach the day of their performance. By knowing their bodies well, and with a great deal of experience, they learn to modify their workout in order to achieve peak performance at the right time. For long distance runners, they will usually stop pushing themselves the week prior to a big race and do mostly gentle jogging, walking and stretching exercises. For football players, intense practice stops prior to the day before the game. Muscles respond by being pushed to their maximum, but they need time to recover. Excessive muscle soreness or minor injuries will impede their performance.

Read on and you will learn how many different exercise techniques can fit into your life.

Chapter 6 – Exercise Techniques

Make a commitment to stick with your exercise program for the long term before you ever start to sweat the first day. Find something you enjoy and stick with it. Start gradually in order to avoid the pitfalls that may lead to failure. Do this and you will avoid the injuries that can occur from overusing deconditioned muscles. Overusing muscles can result in marked delayed onset muscle soreness or "DOMS". This is a painful, cramping pain that may linger for days in overused muscles and inhibit your exercise program.

Find an enjoyable activity from the start and it will greatly increase your chance of success. If you are dreading the boredom of your routine, chances are you are not going to stick with it. Start your program off on the right foot and work to keep it interesting.

Search for the proper balance in your life and decide how much exercise is too much. Look at your goals and ask yourself, "Why am I exercising?" If you have not set any goals, do it today. The simple act of setting a goal and writing it down will greatly increase your chance of success. If exercise in and of itself has become the prime motivator, you may need to re-balance your priorities. With the correct perspective, exercise can improve physical and psychological aspects of your life. Too much exercise does not allow time needed for regeneration and interferes in other parts of your life. Too much exercise will also cause wear and tear and not allow you to enjoy the benefits that good health and fitness can bring. Too little exercise erases the cumulative cardio-pulmonary and strength benefits that are only seen if exercise is done consistently..

Goals made, based on needs and interests will guide what exercises you do. The great UCLA basket ball coach John Wooden said "failure to plan is planning to fail" Make a plan and stick to it. Your personal characteristics, including body habitus, as well as your performance needs will direct your plan.

If you desire to have more cardio-pulmonary endurance, you should do more aerobic activities such as running, bicycling or swimming. If your goal is to improve your performance in a specific sport, you will need to perform sport-specific activities. Evaluate supporting muscles that will help you to perform better. For example, strengthening your legs may help you to hit a tennis ball harder because it gives you a better base of support. Improve your basketball game by working on your balance. In every instance, evaluate your routine and make sure it is consistent with your needs and goals.

Maintain your target heart rate to realize your desired cardiovascular benefits. For a healthy person, this is in the range of seventy to eighty-five percent of your maximum heart rate. Calculate this by subtracting your age from 220 and multiplying that number by 70% to 85%, (220 – your age) x (0.7-0.85). Sustain this heart rate for 30-60 minutes four times per week to improve your condition. Obviously, just remaining active and doing things such as yard work will help to maintain your fitness level but it would not greatly increase a healthy person's cardiopulmonary performance.

Improving your cardiovascular fitness allows your body to be more efficient. Your resting heart rate will be slower and you will have a greater reserve to draw upon to improve your performance. Your ability to consume oxygen, or VO2 max, will increase as well. This is a factor that often separates elite athletes from average competitors. Further, in response to your body's increased performance and blood flow demands, you will actually grow new collateral blood vessels. They will increase the delivery of oxygen and nutrients throughout your body and assist with the removal of the byproducts of exercise.

Aerobics are a popular class of exercises that combine dance, stepping and calisthenics to efficiently burn energy. You work many large muscle groups that all require a great deal of blood flow and oxygenation. The addition of arm movements with or without light weights adds additional toning and strengthening to the aerobic benefit of these classes

Low-impact aerobics decrease your chance of injury and are a desirable choice for exercise because you are able to burn a great deal of energy with less trauma to your body. By utilizing multiple different muscles, you can tone and strengthen your body, providing a "body sculpting" effect while receiving the cardiopulmonary benefit. The need to simultaneously contract specific muscles provides a strengthening effect and a base for other muscles that are working in a sustained, aerobic fashion.

Variety in our exercise routine is essential. Provide time for socialization, games, cross-training or whatever it takes to hold your interest in order to continue exercising over the long run.

Make your exercise fun and it will only multiply your benefits. If you have become bored with your treadmill, run outside. Find some good scenery. Breathe some fresh air. Once running starts to feel too much like work, grab your bike and hit the trails. Most communities have designated bike trails. Try joining an exercise class. In a social setting such as this, you can push and inspire each other to do better. Do whatever it takes to hold your interest. The benefits of exercise are cumulative and, when interrupted by periods of boredom or disinterest, the benefits are lost faster than they were obtained.

Vary your activities and you will achieve multiple skills. If you play tennis, bike, swim, or run as part of your exercise routine, these activities will provide you with skills that will benefit you in other competitive or social situations. Further, you will increase the number of interesting life-long activities that you will be able to do throughout your adult life. Vary your activities and it will avoid overuse injuries that occur when a specific activity is done repeatedly.

The ability to do a variety of different exercises provides the flexibility to adapt your exercise routine to multiple situations. If you are traveling, you may be able to use the hotel gym or run on the city streets. On vacation, you could swim in the pool or ocean if you took the time to learn how to swim. An hour of singles tennis with a friend may count for your usual 30 minute run. The possibilities are endless.

Alternate periods of rest with high and low intensity exercise routines because it is essential to feel your best and perform at your highest level. Periods of intense exercise are necessary to improve speed and strength but these must be balanced with periods of rest to provide time for healing. Fitness is a measure of your overall physical health. To be healthy, adequate rest is essential.

How much rest is needed is going to be different for everyone. It is important that you are in tune to clues your body is giving you about your fitness. Experience will tell you if the fatigue you are feeling is due to poor condition or a need for rest. If you find yourself needing to rest while doing simple household chores, you may need to work to get yourself into better shape. If however you are a long distance runner and you begin to find yourself catching frequent colds or your performance declines, you may be pushing yourself too hard and you simply need more rest.

Walking is a great exercise choice for the simple fact that it is available whenever you are. It offers many advantages, most important being the fact that no equipment is required. No matter what you are wearing, if you have the time, you can go for a walk at work or home. At work I often see two ladies walking briskly around the hospital during their lunch break. They change their shoes, but even that is not absolutely necessary. Obviously the quality of your walking will affect your results but the bottom line is, just get moving! Increase the number of steps you take during the day and you will see great benefits.

To increase the benefits of walking, pay attention to the quality of your walking. Hold your shoulders back and your stomach in. This will improve your posture and strengthen your stomach muscles. Swing your arms to burn more calories and strengthen your upper extremities. Pay attention to heel strike, toe off and all the components of your gait cycle to maximize your results.

Stretching is an essential component of warming up and cooling down before and after strenuous activities. You will perform better, incur fewer injuries, and decrease delayed onset muscle soreness or "DOMS". Rather than jumping right into intense physical activity, take the time to warm up. Walk and then jog before you run. Lift light weights before lifting heavy weights. Warming up will increase the blood flow to the muscles that you will need to use. After you warm up, gently stretch the muscles, tendons and ligaments that you will be using to perform your exercise.

There are two acceptable methods of stretching. In the first method, slowly move to the end of the range of motion of the part of the body you are stretching. Hold it there for a few seconds but do not bounce! You may feel some slight burning pain. With the second method, move to the end point and quickly recede before a muscle stretch reflex is initiated. You can perform both methods independently or with a partner.

Sneaking exercise into your daily routine can be an essential component of any exercise philosophy. Our lives are simply too busy to dedicate hours every day to exercise. The solution is that you do not have to do all of your exercise at once as long as multiple activities add up to the minimum requirement of at least thirty minutes a day, five days a week. Where you park can add many steps to the total you take during a day. Rather than driving around the parking lot, park further away and spend the time briskly walking into the store. Take the stairs instead of the elevator and you will receive strength and aerobic benefits. Isometric exercises can also be done while you are working without interrupting your schedule. While at your desk, tighten and hold muscles of your legs, butt, stomach, arms or neck. You will have gotten in a workout with nobody noticing.

Exercise cost averaging is my modification of the "Pay yourself first" concept. When it comes to investing money for the future, financial planners say that an initial portion of the money you make each day should go to financing your future before you pay other people or your bills. Look at exercise and your health the same way. Carve out time in your day to exercise and make it a priority if you want to accumulate lifelong benefits.

Just like other expenses, many things will come along that will consume our time and leave none left for exercise. This is why it pays to exercise first before you go to work, out to eat, or watch TV, etc. Further, if you exercise consistently, no matter what the situation, you will reap consistent benefits that average out but continue to grow over time and in spite of different demands.

Perspective in all you do is essential. If you realistically examine your exercise goals and persevere through difficult times, you have found the keys to success. Maintain a positive attitude and it will help push you through the times when you do not feel like exercising. Ultimately, exercise needs to be an important part of your life.

You can easily identify people who have a positive attitude towards exercise and who believe that it is important. From their perspective, exercise is as important as many other things they do during the day. They do not look at exercise as work or a chore but an integral part of their day that they could not do without. People who have integrated exercise into their behavior patterns find it hard to stray for long from exercise routines.

I cannot overstate the fact that personal goals should guide any exercise philosophy. These goals should be age appropriate and directed towards maximum benefit and injury prevention. For a non-competitive athlete, contact sports may not be appropriate because of the inherent risk of injury. Placing your livelihood or personal relationships at risk is not worth the cost.

Continually challenge yourself though and it will pay off. Although speed and reflexes are known to decrease as we age, much of the decrease is due to disease rather than advancing years. If you continue to do activities that require strength, speed and agility, you will find that you can maintain these abilities until an advanced age.

Exercise philosophies vary from author to author and among coaches or trainers. Keep asking questions and be a student of exercise. The medical profession is an invaluable resource of knowledge about what you can safely do to improve your health and performance. Research and evaluate the equipment you use and it will enlighten you to new technologies that provide a competitive edge.

New technologies related to exercises, equipment or strategies are always emerging. The PX-90 program has recently become a popular program designed to increase strength and performance. With any program or philosophy, proper exercises done using the right equipment with sound underlying strategies are the recipe for success. Do not be afraid to try new things and incorporate them into your routine. The resources related to diet, exercise and exercise equipment are endless.

Read on and you will learn how to maximize your performance

Chapter 7 – Maximum Performance

Power, simply defined, is the capacity or ability to act. To achieve maximum performance, you need to strive to create the greatest amount of force over the longest distance in the least amount of time. To act with greater effectiveness, athletes break down the individual aspects of power and analyze each one for any deficits. To improve their performance, they focus on every aspect of creating power.

To create more power, you need to apply more force. To improve the force aspect of the equation, you need to increase strength. This occurs through weight lifting or other resistance exercises. Improving performance however, requires that you be able to create this force faster. Speed exercises are therefore essential. To take the next step and be able to perform at a high level, you need to be able to sustain this activity for a period of time and over a significant distance. Learn to create maximum force quickly and maintain it over a significant distance it will enable you to maximize your performance.

VO_2 max, or how much oxygen you are able to consume ultimately, determines how much work you are able to do. Improve your aerobic capacity and strengthen the muscles that you need to carry you through these activities to increase your VO2 max. For each one of us, there is an absolute limit, based on our genetics, to the amount of oxygen we can consume. Oxygen use is what sustains us during prolonged endurance activities. The majority of time, our activities is fueled by oxygen.

Endurance athletes strive for the ability to maximize their consumption of oxygen. For someone like Lance Armstrong, his unique cardiopulmonary system enables him to use far more oxygen than the average person. He needs to simply strengthen his musculoskeletal system enough to realize his VO$_2$ max, VO$_2$ max is made up of your stroke volume, or how much blood your heart pumps, your heart rate and how much oxygen is extracted from your blood (arterial-venous difference). Aerobic exercise improves all components of this equation.

Consistent exercise will help you to maintain maximum performance. Once you've reached a high plain of performance, it is easier to stay there than to have a significant fall-off and then try to repeatedly regain your form. Unfortunately, functional losses occur faster than gains and you cannot afford to take too much time off. Beyond one week, you will notice a significant decline in performance if you have remained sedentary.

If you continuously attempt maximum performance at one specific activity, however, you will pay a physical price. If you are a marathon runner and all you do is long distance running every day, it will take a toll on your body. The practice of cross training is beneficial to both improve performance and decrease injuries. To avoid these overuse injuries and to maintain your performance during periods of recovery from injury, vary your routine. This will further avoid the losses in strength and endurance that occur if you simply rest during a period of recovery or during a break in your routine.

Pushing your muscle to its limit is necessary to achieve significant gains in performance. The breakdown that occurs when pushed close to failure triggers a build up in size and strength in a muscle. For athletes who depend on maximum size and strength, this part of their exercise routine is essential. Body builders need to push their weight lifting to failure nearly every time they lift weights.

For the casual athlete, the desire to add size and strength needs to be balanced against the need to avoid injury. Again, you need to examine your goals when planning your exercise routine. There are more subtle and safer ways to push a muscle to its limit besides heavy weight lifting. Lower weight, high repetition resistance exercises are the most common safe alternative. You may not achieve as much muscle size benefit but you can greatly improve your muscle tone in this manner.

Isolate individual muscles for specific training to further enhance your performance. Tax the same muscles from different angles and with different exercises to develop them further. To achieve greater abdominal muscle tone and strength, do sit-ups with your arms and legs held in different positions and make them burn. Use good form and it will help develop your muscles in a way consistent with how they are going to be used. It will maximize your outcome and avoid injury and make your muscles highly functional from different angles.

Use good form with your exercises and you will create a muscle memory that will be called on unconsciously when needed for activities. It will maximize your performance and create appropriate strength, balance and posture. Challenge and tax your muscles from different angles you will create the strength, stability and agility you need to perform at your best and avoid injury.

Heredity plays a large role in determining at what activities you will excel. Specific exercises however, can change the composition of your body. If you do primarily aerobic activities, you will develop more slow-twitch, oxidative fibers. Because of this, you will excel at endurance activities. If you do more anaerobic exercises, you will develop more fast-twitch fibers and improve your speed.

Anaerobic activities happen more frequently and produce short bursts of force. They draw upon energy sources that can be used faster than oxygen. Aerobic activities require oxygen for sustained function. An example of this can be found in a bird's breast where oxidative processes fuel its ability to fly long distances. If it stopped flying, you would see atrophy of the muscle fibers as well as a smaller proportion of slow-twitch fibers.

The American College of Sports Medicine recommends weight training for all adults. Resistance training is an essential component of any exercise routine and it is universally available. You should try to work it into any aerobic program you are doing. Strengthen your body and you will benefit from a significant protective effect. In the knee, for example, strengthen the thigh and hamstring muscles above the knee and the calf muscles below the knee to stabilize the knee and help avoid injury. Improved Muscle strength and balance around a joint further diminishes the wear and tear within the joint. A portion of the force is absorbed through the soft tissue instead of the joint surface. If present, chronic instability or imbalance will cause multiple small injuries that accelerate the degenerative process. Even if you are an endurance athlete, add weight training to your routine to improve your performance and add longevity to your career. It will add the strength you need to call on during a primarily aerobic activity and prevent injury.

Cardiovascular fitness is an essential component of achieving maximum performance. As previously mentioned, an accurate way of gauging your cardiovascular exertion is the commonly used Max HR equation of 0.7-0.85 x (220 – your age). This gives you a range in which you need to maintain your heart rate while exercising. Perceived exertion however, is a surprisingly accurate way of gauging the amount of work you are doing. The Borg Scale of Perceived Exertion is a classic ordinal scale that translates well to heart rate increase and amount of oxygen consumption.

The Borg Scale is scored from 6-20. It begins with "very, very light" at the bottom to "very, very hard" at the top. If you maintain your exertion at the "hard" level, you should achieve an aerobic training effect. At the hard level, speaking in full sentences will be difficult. Exercise in the "light range and you will still burn calories and improve strength but you won't see a significant aerobic training benefit. For maximum performance benefits, individualize your aerobic program to include the muscle groups necessary for vocational and recreational goals. A generic ergometer or treadmill routine will not meet everyone's needs.

Allowances for recovery must be built into your training schedule. As you age, the speed of recovery will slow. Listen to your body and engage in exercise that you can sustain throughout your life. Over training is a very real phenomenon. The intensity of your exercise needs to vary in order to allow recovery and to achieve your maximum performance.

Muscles respond to loads placed upon them. They grow larger, stronger and more efficient. This process takes time however, and as we age it is slower. Cross training, mentioned earlier accomplishes this result through multiple different activities. You simultaneously build up some muscles while breaking others down. Competitive athletes are always mindful of this as they approach the time at which they need to be at peak performance. They need to make sure that they are not early in their recovery period at a time when they need to be at their best. It is important for everyone to evaluate their goals. If you are an older, weekend athlete you need to be reasonable in your activities. Exercise done too intensely, without a balanced approach, can actually detract from your vocational and physical performance.

Isolate and strengthen specific weaknesses and it will help you achieve maximum performance. Sometimes it takes a trained professional to examine you and test specific muscles. These are weak links that are at risk for injury and affect the performance of your whole body. Once correctable problem areas are identified, a training program can be established.

Specific problem areas may be too strong or too weak, too loose or too tight. A specific example of this is the quadriceps hamstring strength ratio. They are antagonistic muscles that move a joint in the opposite direction. Ideally, their strength ratio should be approximately 3:2. Most commonly, quadriceps will be too strong related to your weaker hamstrings. This occurs frequently because of the natural tendency to work the muscles we can see in the front of our bodies. You should also closely analyze their flexibility. For agonist-antagonist muscles to function well, their degree of flexibility has to be similar. This will allow proper balance and improve performance.

Energy storage ability greatly affects performance over a longer period of time. Build muscle mass and you will increases energy storage capacity. It will provide a reserve of strength and glycogen which can be called upon for strength and endurance.

It is no coincidence that over the years, as world class sprinters have become faster, they have also become more muscular. More muscle mass increases the energy reserve and provides the needed strength and stability joints need to function at their peak level. This strength and energy reserve results in less wear and tear on joints and decreases short term injuries as well as long term degeneration. Increased strength and muscle provides a buffer of extra energy and strength that we can call upon for peak performance.

The good news is that we have the capacity to stay strong until late in life. Disuse is the number one reason for loss of strength and performance capacity, not aging. The saying "use it or lose it" has proven to be true. Based solely on physiological factors, the first noticeable drop off in strength in men does not occur until age 62. This may be related to a slight decrease in testosterone levels more so than anything else.

The media is full of examples of people who have remained strong and fit far beyond their youthful years. Jane Fonda, Sylvester Stallone and Arnold Swartzenegger are prime examples. All of them continue to exercise regularly with resistance and aerobic exercises. Their results are astounding. They demonstrate, clearly, the benefits of a life-long commitment to fitness. Jack Lalane is another prime example of the power of resistance exercises. He remains fit and strong in his mid 90's! Although he started on a plane few people have ever reached, he still looks better than most men sixty years younger than him.

Be consistent with your diet and exercise because it is the key to long term health. Make a point of doing aerobic activities that raise your heart rate to at least 80% of maximum three times a week. If you do this, you will receive many cardiovascular and endurance benefits. At a minimum, just stay active. Simple walks or yard work done on a regular basis help to keep you fit and strong

Cardiovascular exercise should always be done with a goal in mind. If you want to stay active, do regular, low intensity exercise around the house and yard and it will provide impressive results. Along with improved endurance and aerobic capacity, you will be stronger and less prone to injury.

Cross country skiing is the one activity most often cited as providing maximum aerobic benefit. While skiing, you use your legs in a reciprocating motion, your trunk to brace and stabilize your body and your arms to push the poles into the snow. In this activity, you use virtually every large muscle group. Large muscle groups require more blood flow to transport the oxygen they need and remove the byproducts of their work. The heart is challenged over time to provide the needed circulation and it will become stronger and more efficient.

Swimming is another activity that provides great aerobic benefits. By its nature, swimming requires constant, sustained activity. Devoted swimmers develop impressive endurance. Swimming also strengthens your body because it uses multiple muscles of the body simultaneously. It does it in an unloaded, buoyant environment placing less wear and tear on your joints.

Add bursts of speed to your endurance activities to boost performance. These may consist of sprints or "intervals" done during your endurance training. This will increase your success in competitions that require interval bursts of speed. Running full speed for 50 yards every half mile or swimming full speed every tenth lap could achieve this goal.

Sport-specific activities are the final piece needed to maximize your performance. Strength, flexibility and endurance are the initial components. In order to achieve success in a specific sport, you have to uniquely apply these components to your specific sport. By doing so, your muscles will achieve muscle memory. Patterns become engrained in our neuromusculoskeletal system when we repeat them over time. Use good mechanics and the proper technique when training. To be successful at swinging a golf club or pitching a baseball, practice a consistent swing and the proper motion.

Cross training is an important final component of maximum performance. Do activities that add strength or improve balance and endurance and it will help your performance. It further has the benefit of taxing your system in different ways helping to prevent overuse activities. Many competitive athletes have turned to unrelated endeavors such as martial arts or even ballet to improve their performance. For lifelong health and fitness, examine the activities you do and always look for new ways to stay fit for life.

In the following chapter, I discuss an epidemic that has been sweeping our nation and one that affects every age group.

Chapter 8 – Obesity

A body mass index (BMI) greater than 30 defines obesity. Obesity has been called an epidemic in our country because a higher percentage of people in the United States exceed this level than in previous generations. Recently it has begun to be seen more commonly in much younger age groups. Body mass index is your weight in relation to your height. To calculate your BMI, take your weight in pounds and multiply it by 713, then divide it by your height in inches twice. A BMI greater than 30 is considered obese with the ideal range being 18.5-27. Use this number as a relative guide because factors such as increased muscle mass will also increase your BMI without making you obese.

Obesity has begun to receive as much attention as other health risk factors for many reasons. Obesity is linked to elevated cholesterol, blood pressures and blood sugars. These are risk factors for a variety of diseases such as heart disease and stroke. The immobility and arthritis it causes or exacerbates are quality of life issues. The epidemic of obesity has further led to the alarming increase in Type 2 Diabetes or what we used to call Adult-Onset Diabetes".

Technology has brought great prosperity to American society. With it however, has come obesity. Automation of much of what we used to do by hand allows us to burn less calories doing what we need to do to get through the day. With the surpluses that most of us enjoy however, our calorie intake has not declined accordingly.

Simply getting through the day a hundred years ago required a great deal of effort and physical exertion. People would wash their clothes by hand. They would hunt and gather food in order to feed their families. Rarely was there extra food around the house to eat. Further, they did not drive to work or take an elevator when they got there. When they got to work, most likely it consisted of physical farming or assembly work. There was no way for them to avoid constant physical activity.

Genetic makeup of human beings has remained relatively constant for generations. Because of our free will and higher consciousness, we are resistant to the evolutionary forces placed upon the rest of the plant and animal kingdoms. What has changed is our environment. The so-called "thrifty gene" which better enabled people to store fat and conserve energy during times of want was a great survival asset in the past. Today however, this instinct leads to obesity. We appear programmed to overeat due to generations in which periods of great hunger existed. In America today, food is bountiful and relatively inexpensive. Couple this with an environment that asks little from us physically to survive and it is no wonder we are overweight.

It is ironic that what enabled you to survive generations ago may be killing you now. Energy intake versus output needs to be re-balanced. To do this, make an honest assessment of consumption and energy burned throughout the day.

Donuts versus bagels. Chips versus celery. Beer or pop versus water. These and many more choices like these present themselves throughout your day and can have a significant impact on your weight. These are choices that you make as you pass through the grocery aisles, drive up to a fast food window or stand in front of your refrigerator.

Do not waste calories. I am not saying to never indulge in some junk food occasionally. But if you do, make it worth it. If you never indulge in treats, you will feel that you are making a sacrifice and this will adversely effect how you feel about eating healthy. If someone bakes a fresh fruit pie, by all means, have a piece. Life is too short to pass it by. But if there is an old donut available that has been sitting out all day, don't eat it just because it is there. You will feel lousy anyway. When you are looking for a snack, make a healthy choice every time. Stop and ask yourself if you are truly hungry or just bored. Make it easier to make the right choice by having fruits and vegetables around the house and office.

Television has had a negative effect on the fitness of American society. For every hour of T.V. that a child averages per day, obesity rises 6%. This is due to more than just the fact that a child is not outside running around when he or she is watching TV. Commercials flood our minds with colorful and inviting images of unhealthy foods and drinks. Children in particular are vulnerable to these images and they affect their eating habits as well as what they ask their parents to buy.

Because television is so passive, few activities burn fewer calories. There is decreased metabolic activity of our minds and bodies. It is significantly less than other quiet activities such as reading. The television tends to interrupt your natural inclination to move slightly while doing sedentary activities. What little activity that is triggered is usually unhealthy. While we are burning minimal calories, we are simultaneously being encouraged to eat unhealthy foods.

Inexpensive snacks flood grocery store shelves and refrigerators throughout our homes and workplace. Processed foods are so plentiful because they have been created to last longer. During the preservation process, much of the beneficial textures and nutrients are lost. They have been packaged to be convenient and they are cheap.

Fresh, healthy foods, by their nature, will not last as long as processed foods. This makes it even more important to take the time to have more healthy choices available. You will need to shop more often for smaller quantities. Schools and institutions need to change how they store and present choices. It is a cultural change but it could begin with simple things like providing trays of cut carrots or broccoli.

The quality and quantity of food we consume has changed significantly over the past generation. Portion size has increased by 30-40%. Weight Watchers has had great success with their clients by simply teaching them the importance of decreasing their portion size. Hormones fed to livestock have been implicated in the ever-expanding size of Americans. Genetic modification of produce has improved the visual appeal and increased the disease resistance of fruits and vegetables but it has decreased their nutrient content. In spite of this food remains relatively inexpensive.

Although relatively cheap, the least expensive foods are frequently not the most nutrient rich. They are frequently full of preservatives, fats and simple sugars and lack fiber and nutrients. The ability to easily ingest a large quantity of calorie dense, high fat, high sugar foods quickly before our natural satiety mechanism has time to trigger us to stop further increases the risk of obesity.

The fundamental issue with regards to weight loss is that you must burn more calories than you consume. You need to balance your input versus output to maintain your weight. To lose weight, you need to tip the scale in favor of output. Calorie dense, unhealthy foods make it more difficult to do this

To tip the scale, you need to either decrease your intake or increase your output. Small decreases in intake throughout the day can have huge cumulative benefit. A small, 200 calorie cookie would require thirty minutes of walking briskly to burn off. So make your calories worth it. On the other hand, if you choose to tip the scale by increasing your energy expenditure, a significant amount of healthy food is required as fuel for energy or to build muscle.

The time it takes to control our intake and to prepare healthy food makes eating healthy more difficult. Set the time aside and make it a priority to eat healthy. Fresh food takes time to prepare and has a shorter shelf life than preserved, calorie-dense food. Most of the prepared, convenient, microwavable foods are unhealthy. It is ironic that as we take less time to prepare and eat our meals, we are actually eating more calories. Lost in this is the richness of the experience of preparing and cooking your own food. The convenience of prepared foods has tricked us into unhealthy habits.

Temptations exist everywhere that can derail the best diet plans. Everyone is susceptible to caving into unhealthy habits. Certain steps must be taken to reduce the temptations. For starters, do not bring the unhealthy food into your home. If it is there, chances are you will eat it. When you feel hungry, the unhealthy food may seem like the best option. If you bought it, you may just not want it to go to waste. Also, do not shop hungry. You will find that you come home with too many items that provide instant gratification but little nutritional value.

Associated behaviors further reinforce unhealthy eating. If you tend to eat a lot of junk food every time you watch television, you may need to change your TV schedule. Frequent restaurant dining as well may make it more difficult to eat healthy. Most menus are filled with large-portion, calorie-dense offerings. Applebees has begun to advertise 500 calorie entrees. I think they are on to something. This is about half of what normal restaurant entrées contain. Look for behaviors that are associated with healthy eating. In general, it is always a safe bet to substitute physical activity for an unhealthy habit.

The reward for a healthy lifestyle is lifelong health benefits. Temporary effects are rarely relevant. Athletes may diet to achieve a desired wrestling weight class temporarily. A body builder may cut his calories significantly right before a competition. He does this for temporary visual discrimination of his muscles for a competition. For the average person, temporary changes in behavior are not healthy and should not be the goal.

Do not diet. Change your life. Dieting has too many negative connotations and implies a temporary behavior change. In order to be healthier and happier, make food and activity choices that enable you to sustain an ideal weight for the rest of your life. Establishing your own personal "set point" is healthier and easier to maintain than wide metabolic fluctuations caused by large changes in diet and activity. Make your personal "set point" be your target that you shoot for with balanced diet and exercise

The weight we carry will in large measure affect the way we move through life and. If you are fit and well-conditioned, you will move through daily activities with energy to spare. Our overall well-being is tied closely to our physical condition and impacts the quality of our lives. If we are in better shape and eating right, we will have more energy and be more efficient.

If you have significant energy reserves, energy needed to do self care tasks or transferring ourselves will be drawn from our reserves and not deplete energy needed for vocational or recreational activities. For extremely obese or disabled people, simply moving throughout their homes and caring for themselves uses all of their available energy.

The fact that there is food everywhere makes weight loss and weight maintenance all the more difficult. You need to be constantly vigilant of the attacks on your waistline. Workplaces are frequently awash with junk food placed at easily accessible locations. High fat or high sugar items such as donuts are usually the easiest to find.

Our modern society does many things that makes weight loss difficult and has contributed to the obesity epidemic. Driving, not walking, down the road, fast food is everywhere. Morgan Spurlock, in his movie "Supersize Me," talked of the adverse effects that fast food has had on the health of our society. He took it a step further and ate nothing but fast food for a month to demonstrate the dramatic and frightening effects it has on your body. The high calorie content and ready availability are a deadly combination.

Cravings occur in response to metabolic imbalances as well as subtle psychological cues and can sabotage any good diet plan. The good news is that they can be markedly reduced over time with a healthy diet and exercise. Balanced diets with high macrobiotic content will damper the wild blood sugar fluctuation that may lead to carb cravings. As you become accustomed to a diet of high quality foods, a diet of high fat, high sodium choices will grow unappealing.

Adjust your intake over time to a lower calorie, balanced diet and it will allow you to slowly lose weight. You do not have to feel hungry all the time. When David Letterman moved his show to 11:30, and walked into Johnny Carson's bright spotlight, he made a point of losing weight. He said that he went to bed hungry every night. This worked for him temporarily but did not become his permanent habit. Long term, this is not a good plan for weight maintenance. Low-calorie, high bulk, nutrient-rich foods can simultaneously allow you to lose weight while satisfying your hunger.

Obesity matters because of the cost to society as well as the personal costs. Large amounts of additional healthcare resources are needed because of obesity. These include treatment of the associated cardiac and musculoskeletal diseases and other related conditions. This is relevant today as the debate over the cost of healthcare reform and personal responsibility heats up. Diet and exercise can positively affect most disease states decreasing the need for or improving the effectiveness of their expensive medical or surgical treatments.

Obesity matters also because of the associated waste with excessive consumption. I tip my hat to vegetarians who eat food that is taken directly from the earth, bypassing the need to feed and raise animals and deal with their waste. The amount of material resources used to raise animals to make super sized value meals is astounding when compared to the environmental cost of simply growing something and eating it directly.

In the next chapter, I present an alternative goal that will provide great health benefits.

Chapter 9 - Tone

Safety is a major benefit of training for "tone" instead of strength. This relates to both unintended accidents that may occur when lifting heavy weights as well as the cumulative injuries that still occur when everything is done correctly. Avoid the wear and tear of repetitive high intensity workouts on your joints and it will provide long term benefits. Personal appearance is one of the primary reasons people do specific toning exercises. This is particularly true for people who want to project a youthful, healthy appearance more so than building large muscles.

High repetitions of lower weight exercises results in firming and toning of muscles. It will not cause as much hypertrophy of muscles as loading a muscle with maximum force. But by doing so, you can still achieve strength and performance benefits but at a lower risk. Potential injuries from using maximum force with exercise include disc herniations, muscle and tendon pulls or even hernias. For the non-competitive athlete or average person, the risk of maximum force training greatly outweighs the benefits. A weak link exists in everyone's body, and if you continue to exert maximal force, you will find it.

Consistent effort will enable you to address and get rid of problem areas. Analyze the basic muscle function of the problem area and it will direct you to the types of toning exercises you should do. Give specific attention to these areas to receive the desired benefit. Consider the functions of the muscles that support your low back, for example, and it will guide an exercise routine that can tone and shrink your waistline

If you are not seeing the changes you expected, analyze the specific areas and modify your routine to affect the change. You may need to increase you repetitions and push your muscles more to the point of fatigue. You may need to attack the area from different angles. In most cases, your body will adapt by toning the specific areas. This can have multiple benefits including improved appearance as well as injury prevention in that region.

Attack muscles from different angles and it will allow you to apply more work to a muscle and exercise it to its full capacity. A joint's range of motion and its functional paths of motion will increase. Muscle function in multiple different positions and its overall tone will improve. Weight machines that work muscles different ways or mat exercises are both ideal ways to accomplish this.

Exercise muscles from different angles and you will receive multiple performance and injury-prevention benefits. Our muscles are asked to do work in a variety of positions and angles while competing. The stronger and more flexible we are, the better we will perform. For large muscles such as the abdominals, the performance benefits of exercising them from different angles will be even more rapidly realized.

Eccentric contractions are muscle contractions that occur as the muscle is lengthening. In strength training, they are referred to as "negatives." Slightly more work is done by a muscle contracting eccentrically that has been maximally loaded than a muscle that is shortening while lifting maximum weight. To do negatives correctly, slowly allow your muscle to lengthen in a controlled manner.

Negatives can be safer than traditional lifting because you are avoiding the jerking activity of a maximal lift. This eliminates sudden increases in force on tendons, ligaments and muscles as well as intra-abdominal or thoracic pressure. Because you are loading your muscles steadily during an eccentric contracture, you are strengthening it at every joint angle. As a note of caution, you may initially notice more delayed onset muscle soreness as you add them to your workout regimen because of the consistent load placed upon your muscles.

Walking is a perfect time to work on abdominal tone. Tighten your stomach muscles when you walk and you will efficiently improve your abdominal tone. Sitting is another opportunity to exercise your abdominals. Hold your stomach muscles in while you are sitting and you will achieve long term benefits with regards to your stomach tone. You may notice an added benefit of your back feeling better because you are bracing your spine. Do abdominal exercises in bed first thing in the morning as an easy way to fit them into your day.

Ideal positioning for abdominal exercises is a 90-90 posture with your hips and knees both flexed to 90 degrees. You can then put both your hands behind your ears and do partial sit-ups or "crunches." To tone your lower abdominal muscles on the sides, roll partially one way and then direct the force of your sit-up to the opposite hip. Lie on your back and do a bicycle motion or use a device such as a "Thera Ball" to tone and strengthen your stomach if crunches become tiresome. The "Thera Ball" adds additional toning because you need to control the rolling motion of the all in all directions.

Take the stairs instead of the elevator during the day to tone and strengthen your thighs. It does more than burn calories and improve cardiovascular condition. Perform squats with weight placed on your shoulders and going from full extension to 90 degrees flexion to greatly increase your thigh strength. Do leg presses in a gym on a weight machine as a safer way to add strength and tone to your upper legs. Insert these exercises into your day. The possibilities are endless!

To perform closed kinetic chain thigh exercises, anchor your feet against the ground or the foot plate of a piece of exercise equipment. This is a safer, more physiologic and beneficial means of doing toning exercises. They require much more coordinated activity between muscles and joints and are more consistent with how we usually use our leg exercises. Open kinetic chain thigh exercises allow your feet to swing freely. An example of this is a knee extension machine commonly found in your local gym.

Strengthen and tone your gluteal muscles by performing hip extension exercises. With our feet touching the ground, we use these muscles as we stand erect from a flexed position. With our feet floating freely, hip extension occurs when you bend your leg backwards while lying face down, or pronated, with your knees out straight. The smaller gluteus medius and minimus which are located more laterally are used primarily for hip abduction. To exercise these muscles, swing your legs out away from your midline. This can be done while lying on your back or side. To do "glute" sets means to isometrically contract your gluteal muscles or buttocks, while sitting or lying on your back.

Strengthen and tone your gluteal muscles because they form an essential part of your foundation. Your performance depends upon a good foundation and base of support. This applies to arm activities such as throwing a ball as well as leg activities such as running.

Adduct your shoulders by exercises such as "butterflies" to strengthen and tone your chest muscles. Butterflies are done with weights held in both hands lying on your back. Start with your arms out to your sides and carefully bring the weight to your midline in front of your chest. Bench presses, doing elbow extensors while lying on your back, also works your chest muscles. Do abductor stretches to avoid shortening of your shoulder adductors. To do this, stand in a doorway with your hand on the frame, lean forward and passively take your arm back to the end of its range with your elbow extended.

Stretch your chest muscles and strengthen the upper back muscles to provide balance for proper shoulder function and to avoid pain and injury. Add exercises that retract your shoulders when doing a chest strengthening program. Rowing exercises pull your shoulders back and create this desired motion. Perform them on a regular basis and it will avoid the impaired function and undesirable appearance of protracted, drooped shoulders.

To tone your biceps, perform lower weight, higher repetition elbow curls. They are called biceps brachii because they are a two-headed muscle in the anterior portion of your arm. Many weight lifters emphasize them when it comes to exercise because of the high profile they have with regards to appearance. To further tone your biceps, supinate your forearm, turn your palm up, while flexing your elbow and pronate, turn your palm down, while extending your elbow. You will tone both the biceps and the underlying brachialis if you use both techniques with your curls.

Do "negative" or eccentric contractions to further strengthen and tone your biceps. To do so, slowly extend your elbow while holding a weight.

Achieve optimal biceps strength and it will improve many athletic endeavors, such as racquet sports that require strong elbow flexion. Exercise your muscles with higher repetitions and lower weights and it will train them to be more fatigue resistant. The results will shine through in the sixth game of the third set.

Balance of muscle strength, size and length on both sides of the body is critically important. Work on your back muscles is necessary to ensure this balance. A variety of exercises specifically address this issue. Rowing, either on a machine or in a boat strengthens the back extensors muscles that retract and depress your shoulders. Strengthening and toning these muscles is critical to balancing the strong anterior muscles of the chest and arms. For appearance sake, working on your back muscles will improve your posture and balance. From a performance standpoint, strengthening these muscles will improve performance and help to avoid injury.

Balance strength and flexibility in your shoulders. Strengthen the back muscles to avoid common rotator cuff injuries. Our natural inclination is to let our shoulders droop. A major factor in shoulder problems is the long term consequences of holding a position of protracted/anterior shoulders. This places the rotator cuff at a mechanical disadvantage and leads to premature wear and tear. Shoulder shrugs, in addition to the previously mentioned rowing will also strengthen the back muscles to achieve maximum performance and avoid injury.

Tone and strengthen your neck or cervical muscles from a variety of angles. Flex your neck, or bend it forward, and extend it, or bend it backwards. In addition to this, you should add rotation exercises against resistance. Isometric exercises are safely done when a force is applied, and a constant muscle length is maintained. Perform these easily on your own neck by placing your hand on your head and resist flexion, extension or rotation. These are very safe exercises but always remember to exhale with each repetition.

Traction added to your neck strengthening program can have long term benefits. Traction gently distracts the soft tissues of the neck. By doing so, it avoids shortening of the tissues; it provides some pain relief and may even serve to gently withdraw bulging discs. A variety of traction devices exist including, over the door sand or water bags, hydraulic machines, or traction applied by another individual. The best traction devices make contact at the mastoids and forehead, not the jaw, and apply approximately 15-20 pounds of force with the neck flexed 10-15 degrees.

Body fat measurements using skin calipers are taken from the triceps. The amount of adipose surrounding our triceps is a fair indication of our overall body fat. A health professional painlessly pinches the skin behind the triceps and reads a number from the dial. To tone, strengthen and improve the appearance of your arms, body composition needs to be considered. Strengthen your triceps with exercises that extend the elbow. These are frequently done in conjunction with exercises that adduct the shoulder. The bench press is the most common exercise done to strengthen and tone the triceps as well as the chest muscles.

Triceps strength and endurance are essential for many vocational and recreational activities. To push merchandise or tools at work or throw a ball in sports requires fast and strong elbow extension. As we get older, we rely on triceps strength even more to assist with transfers and gait.

Walk regularly to tone and strengthen your calves. The calves are made up of the medial and lateral gastrocnemius and the underlying soleus. They primarily serve to plantar flex your ankle or to "push off." High heeled shoes serve to make calves more attractive by maintaining a contracted position, but they are not good for your feet or your legs. Popular rocker bottom shoes tone and strengthen your legs because they require you to constantly fire multiple leg muscles when walking or standing.

Calf muscles are also important postural stabilizer muscles. They have the highest ratio in the body of muscle fibers to nerves. As such, they are not designed for fine movements. They are intended to help maintain balance and for gait. Heel raises are another way to strengthen your calves. Perform this exercise with your heels suspended and contract your calves to lift your heels.

Strengthen the muscles that surround a joint in order to protect it and decrease wear and tear. Strengthen the muscle and less force is transmitted through the joint itself. Tone and strengthen the muscles around the hip joint to receive many other benefits. Strengthen the hip flexors, extensors, abductors and adductors to improve gait stability and muscle tone. The benefits of good hip strength extend all the way up the spine and assist with a good base of support.

To address the muscles on the sides of your hips, swing your foot away from your body against resistance. For your inner thighs, draw your legs inward like Suzanne Summers demonstrates on the "thigh master" equipment. Hip extension occurs while walking up stairs or lying on your stomach lifting your leg backwards. Hip flexion occurs when you are lying on your back and you kick your leg forward or when you sit up.

Hand muscle tone and strength are essential because the terminal portion of the lever is where the action will occur. Proximal joints and muscles move this lever through space, but your hands are required to do most of the work. The actual strength and movement of your hands is provided by short intrinsic muscles in your hands and long finger movers your forearms. Strengthen and stretch the muscles in both your hands and arms to achieve optimal performance.

Squeeze a ball or another type of grip strengthening device to strengthen the finger flexor muscles of the hand and forearm. The intrinsic muscles of the hand can achieve remarkable force for their size. Abduct, or spread your fingers apart, and adduct, draw them together, and extend your fingers. Perform all of these motions when strengthening your hands. No part of the body should be neglected when toning your muscles.

In the following chapter, I discuss a common condition that can be greatly improved with exercise.

CHAPTER 10 - ARTHRITIS

Exercise is an important means of controlling your arthritis. Strength and flexibility are the two components of an arthritis exercise program. Strengthen the muscles around a joint and more force will be transmitted through the muscles and soft tissues and more of the force will be taken off the joint itself. Flexibility exercises help maintain a joint's range of motion. They further assist with the health of a joint by improving its nutrition and joint fluid status.

Assess what is going to be most beneficial based on the disease process when devising your exercise program. With an inflammatory arthritic process, such as rheumatoid arthritis, isometric strengthening exercises are the most important because they strengthen a diseased joint and diminish the deformities and hypermobility. In osteoarthritis, flexibility exercises are most important to maintain range of motion. Have your doctor confirm through testing which type of arthritis you have.

Arthritic patients frequently have trouble sleeping. They experience restless legs and aching joints frequently after going to bed. Aerobic exercise can help with this by improving circulation to the joints and muscles and by stretching painful joints. You will expend more of your stored energy and feel ready to rest. Burn calories during the day and be active and you will sleep better

Improve your levels of stress hormones, endorphins and serotonin through exercise. These hormones will help you fall asleep, stay asleep and improve your level of well being. From a common sense standpoint, we all know that if you do not do much physically during the day, you just do not feel as tired at night. There is also less clinical depression in people who perform regular aerobic exercise.

Increased stress on joints because of excess weight is a factor that increases the morbidity in arthritis. Maintain an ideal body weight to minimize these excess forces. Although arthritis is usually a progressive disease regardless of body weight, decrease your weight if you are overweight or obese. It will limit the wear and tear and allow optimum function

In some cases, ideal body weight means the difference between being mobile at a modified independent level versus being nearly bed ridden. Modified independence with mobility means that you are able to get around with the use of a device such as a walker or cane. Head off excessive weight gain before it happens. If you have arthritis, this is critical to maintain your mobility. Once you have gained the weight, weight loss exercises are even more difficult if you have painful and stiff joints.

Empowered by the increased strength and energy that exercise provides, arthritic patients will be able to be more active and independent. Your self esteem is elevated and your willingness to participate in their community is improved. To age successfully, you need to be able to maintain your independence as much as possible. Arthritis is a chronic condition that threatens that goal. For those who fight back against arthritis, they find it much easier to function at a high level. Exercise helps you to remain strong and flexible and to prevent the falls that can so commonly rob the elderly of their independence.

Instability of joints is a condition that can both lead to and worsen arthritis. As part of the degenerative cascade, the body's natural response to instability is to provide stability. To do so, the body will produce boney spurs or arthritic changes. As a result, the joints are stiffer and less functional. Instability of a joint caused by trauma, weakness or imbalances needs to be addressed early in this process.

Strengthen muscles on either side of an arthritic joint to stabilize it and diminish the trauma to the joint surface. Some of the force will be absorbed by the stronger muscles. With osteoarthritis, maintain the proper range of motion through stretching exercises to maintain joint balance and stability.

Stretching may be the most important component of your arthritic exercise program. Before beginning, however, see your doctor to help you establish what is right for you. If you have a type of inflammatory arthritis such as rheumatoid arthritis, you may need to do little stretching. Instead, you may need to do primarily strengthening. A thorough exam may determine that you need to do focused stretching. An example of this is the intrinsic or small muscles of the hands, which may shorten with chronic inflammation.

Adequate range of motion, however, is of paramount importance with any patient. Emphasize stretching first to enable yourself to increase strength through the full range of motion. Stretch on a regular basis and not as an immediate precursor to physical activity. In the book, "Stretching" by Bob Anderson, he talks about adding frequent, spontaneous stretches throughout your day. This is far superior to the common practice of just stretching before physical activity.

Cardiovascular exercises are another important component of an exercise program for people with arthritis. A cardiovascular exercise program provides increased endurance that makes it easier to do your needed strengthening exercises. Circulation improves as well with cardiovascular exercise. This improves muscle and joint health. Aerobic, cardiovascular conditioning makes many daily tasks easier.

Being short of breath and in poor cardiovascular condition adds another significant burden to arthritic patients. In pain and with stiff joints, it is tempting to move as little as possible. If you have arthritis, this is the worst thing you can do. You will lose strength and mobility more rapidly than the average person.

Expect muscle soreness and joint tenderness when you begin your exercise program. Start slow and gradually increase the time and intensity of your workouts. Listen to your body and rest when needed. Keep track of your exercise regimen in an exercise log and it will be a great motivational tool as well as you track your progress.

When you exercise, try to be in tune to how your body is reacting. Take your pulse and make sure that it is in a regular rhythm and that you achieve a sustained heart rate elevation. Pay attention to the pain you are having. Is it an aching pain in your muscles the day after exercise or is it severe or stabbing pain associated with redness or swelling of your joints? If you have these symptoms, modify your routine and notify your physician.

Support groups can be a great source of information and motivation. Bringing people together that share common impairments can foster camaraderie and let people know that they don't have to suffer alone. The Arthritis Foundation is one of the largest organizations supporting the arthritis community. It provides education, research and support to people with arthritis. It is a great resource that can be used in many ways.

Support groups can make finding the resources you need much more efficient. Whether it is classes on nutrition and weight maintenance or information on home modifications, they would be able to direct you towards it. The Arthritis Foundation offers exercise programs that are tailored to the group's needs.

Aquatic exercises provide resistance with much less stress applied across the joint. Under water, it is much less painful to move an arthritic joint through its range of motion. The buoyancy of a pool provides the added benefit of diminishing balance deficits. Movements that could not be performed on land are done with relative ease in the water.

For the arthritic patient, an aquatic exercise program may enable you to "float" a painful extremity through the painful points of its range of motion. A warm pool may further help to loosen painful joints and add some degree of pain relief. In the water you can mimic many of the motions done on land such as walking or stair climbing. With the added buoyancy and resistance, significant strength and flexibility gains can be made that transfer to on-land activities. Most communities offer aquatic programs through the Arthritis Foundation, the YMCA or community pools.

Proper body mechanics are essential for arthritic patients. With lifting, it is important to maintain good alignment. Proper body mechanics forbids combined bending and twisting activities and the use of awkward postures. Maintain your body weight over your pelvis and you will avoid most back injuries. In a healthy adult, with relaxed standing, your center of gravity falls 4 cm anterior to your sacrum, at the base of your spine. Arthritic patients have a natural tendency to assume a flexed posture Keep your body weight passing through the correct line with all lifting activities and it will help to maintain good strength and posture and decrease injuries.

Positions in which arthritic patients sit or sleep are important to decrease pain. With sitting, you need to ensure good lumbar support to maintain your normal lumbar lordosis. The height of the seat should be such that your hips and knees are flexed to 90 degrees. When sleeping, whether on your side, stomach or back, maintain your spine in a neutral position, without any abnormal curves. When lying on your side, place a cervical pillow under your neck and a pillow between your knees to accomplish this goal.

Configure your environment in an ergonomic manner to significantly improve your efficiency. For a patient with arthritis, this is critically important. The height at which essential objects or appliances are placed may be the difference between using them or not. Divide objects into lighter components and you will be able to lift and transfer just as much material. In the kitchen, for example, divide a five pound bag of flour into one pound portions. Devices designed to do some basic tasks make the work of an arthritic patient much easier. Many of these simple devices are available to the public through catalogs.

Consult with your doctor or therapist, and they can prescribe activity modifications to make your life easier. Other healthcare providers such as Occupational Therapists stress work simplification to maintain a patient's functional independence and still complete basic tasks. They evaluate essential tasks and provide suggestions on how an arthritic patient can complete them more easily. Home evaluations, offered by many physical rehabilitation units provide individualized advice in the patient's unique environment. These steps may be what it takes to allow the arthritic patient to remain in their own home.

Assistive devices provide a great deal of benefit to an arthritic patient seeking to maintain their independence. A patient using an assistive device is said to be functioning at a modified independent level. With the help of the device, they are able to do all of their activities without another person's help. Assistive devices can decrease the work needed to perform activities of daily living, self care activities and mobility skills. These include bathing dressing, eating, toileting, walking, climbing stairs and transferring.

The biomechanical benefit of a straight cane or walker across a painful joint is remarkable. Your arm holding a cane creates a long lever arm that transfers much of the force to the device and off the painful, arthritic joint. For most patients, this is the hip or knee. A cane provides great stability and decreases the lateral deviation that occurs with hip pain and weakness. For many people, this is the difference between walking and being in a wheelchair.

For the times when you cannot avoid activities, the best way to manage them is to control them. Use slow, deliberate, efficient movements and pace yourself. Take needed breaks and avoid working a muscle to fatigue which may place your arthritic joint at risk.

Specific devices such as reachers help to manage the environment. Reachers can prevent the need to bend below your waist or may enable one to pinch a thin object with the needed force. For dressing, a sock aid is beneficial for an arthritic patient who has had hip surgery and is not allowed to bend past their waist or for a patient with pain or stiffness in their low back. Many other devices exist ranging from simple things to the elaborate. These include long shoe horns, electric lift chairs for people with proximal hip girdle weakness or elaborate environmental control units for quadriplegic patients.

The key or all arthritic patients, is keep moving. Exercise can actually nourish an arthritic joint. A joint that is not moved will eventually become stiff, dry and may eventually fuse. Circulation improves in response to exercise challenges. This improved blood flow will support the joint's health. Pain-causing substances such as lactic acid or nitrous oxide will be more efficiently cleared and you will function better. Synovial fluid or joint fluid is also replenished in response to movement.

Strength and flexibility are the two most important components of an exercise program for people with arthritis. Work with your healthcare professionals, and design a program to maximize both of these components and minimize the amount of disability that results from your arthritic impairment. The key is to keep moving.

In the next chapter you will learn how everyone can fit exercise into their everyday activities.

CHAPTER 11 - EXERCISE WITH EVERYDAY ACTIVITIES

Move through life in an energetic way and it will affect how you look and feel. You will burn more calories and maintain a higher level of fitness. Move slowly at all times and you will burn fewer calories and you will cover less ground. An arthritic patient may need to conserve some movements throughout the day, but their movements should be energetic as well. You can preserve and enable movement late into life if you move correctly today.

How you move through the day affects many aspects of your health and physical performance. You learn what you do and become what you have learned. If you maintain good posture when you walk, you will be a person with good posture. If you use good body mechanics and proper lift techniques with your work activities, you will have less pain and be a more balanced, flexible person.

Elevator or stairs? The choices you make during the day have a profound impact on your life. How you lift objects and to what height may be the difference between injuring your back and working relatively pain-free. Where you park your car determines how much more you walk in a day. The subtle effects of all of these decisions throughout our day contribute greatly to your well-being

You determine your strength and condition and to a certain extent how much pain you have by frequent, small choices that you make throughout the day. The cumulative effect of all these things is better health. Along with better health is better aerobic condition and improved strength.

Make healthy choices and you will realize that they do not use up any more of our time and, after a while, they become automatic.

Mechanization and technology make our lives easier and decrease the need for much of the historical physical exertion. The TV remote, a poster child for the couch potato, is the guiltiest subject. Watch television and you will burn fewer calories than sitting quietly in a chair or reading a book. With the advent of the remote, we do not need to move anything except for our thumb. In our society the average person spends many hours on the computer surfing the internet. These sedentary activities displace much of the time spent on physical activities.

Appliances were invented to simplify our daily tasks but the use of them has unintended consequences. Human beings are the only species to use tools for work. This separates us from lower forms of life. Many of the activities that people many years ago spent all day doing can be done now with a push of a button. When you don't spend your time preparing everything from scratch or washing clothes at a river, there is more time for leisure. Usually this consists of a sedentary activity. The secret is to use your leisure time wisely.

Physical activity, done simultaneously while doing something else can add physical activity to your life. Because you are still doing what needed to be done, the physical movement does not take up any more time. Add slight physical activity while doing something like talking on the phone or reading the paper and you'll notice a difference. You can easily take steps around your house while you are talking to someone.

Daily, formal gym exercise is a luxury that is not reasonable for most busy people. When you are too busy to exercise formally, stay active throughout the day and it will pay great dividends. Park a little farther away; add extra steps to your day; or do gentle stretching while working. It may not make a big difference on the athletic field but it will help to maintain your fitness.

Enjoyable exercises are the best exercises for the simple reason that they are the ones most likely to be done. As good as an exercise may be it does not matter if it is not easily and conveniently performed. To be effective, do your exercises on a regular basis. Only consistent use of a muscle or organ system will improve its performance.

To make exercises more enjoyable you must do what you can to avoid boredom. This may mean putting your exercise bike or treadmill in front of a television or, when possible, actually run or bike outside. If you like to socialize, join an exercise class like jazzercise where you can exercise with friends and motivate each other. Think long-term when beginning a program and try to make it enjoyable to avoid burn out.

Postural exercises can be done throughout the day without anyone even noticing. While standing talking on the phone, you can be tightening your abdominals or actively retract your shoulders. The simple act of walking is another way in which you can add exercise by adding the number of steps you take in a day. Work multiple different muscles specifically and use good body mechanics while lifting to add strength to your whole body.

The cumulative effect of little motions and postures that we do throughout the day has a profound effect on your fitness and body habitus. Simple movements consistently done while completing our daily activities really add up. It is no coincidence that the obesity epidemic has occurred recently in conjunction with automation that has resulted in less active lives.

The cost of formal exercise programs or gyms can be prohibitive for some people. Walking is always free and is one of the most efficient and effective exercises. Carrying and lifting objects correctly throughout the day are also free exercises. Be mindful of your movements and postures. Repetitive use of poor body mechanics and incorrect lift techniques can accelerate degenerative changes or lead to injury and is detrimental. The consistent use of proper lift techniques at work results in a resistance work out by the end of the day. Stretch your muscles frequently because it is another convenient, valuable and free exercise.

To avoid injury, consider the quality of the physical activity that you add to your day. If you stretch, do so gently but consistently. When lifting, use good techniques and do not lift objects that are too large for you based on your size and body habitus. Use your legs as much as possible for any heavy lifts and don't be afraid to decline to lift an object you cannot safely handle

Add fun to your exercise routine to get a good workout without realizing how hard you have worked. Office teams foster fun competition and inspire you to perform at a higher level. Fun physical activity will be scheduled into your calendar. Jogging is fun for outdoor lovers who want to breathe fresh air and pass different scenery. Explore what is fun for you and it will make your exercise enjoyable.

Many people stay fit through a regular schedule of fun activities without formal exercise programs. Children are a model of this habit. When outside, they run, climb, ride bikes and explore their environment. They do these things without consciously thinking about exercise. These fun activities develop their strength, balance, endurance and coordination.

Injuries insert a roadblock to good fitness and should be avoided as their effects will add up over the years. A debilitated person is someone who has suffered multiple small injuries over the years and is deconditioned. The resulting pain and stiffness decreases their musculoskeletal and cardiopulmonary performance in a cumulative manner. "No pain, no gain" is a principle that rarely applies to the average person. In rare cases, it is true when trying to add strength and muscle bulk but you need to be cautious. This refers to muscle soreness and not significant pain that lingers long after the activity.

Muscle bulk and strength is added in response to maximum forces placed upon them. For a body builder with appropriate spotting this may be desirable. For the casual athlete, this involves too much risk. In many cases, pain is a warning sign that should not be ignored. There is a fine line between taxing a muscle or joint to its limit and injury.

Isometric exercises are a contraction of a muscle without joint movement. These can be done throughout the day while in the car, on the phone or at your desk. As an example, you can strengthen your neck muscles while at your desk by pushing your forehead against your hand in a variety of directions while preventing head movement.

Isometrics create the added benefit of providing strengthening without movement. This is useful if you need to strengthen a painful region. If your knee hurts, you can still contract and relax your thigh muscles or push your foot against the floor board of your car. Isometrics provide a means of maintaining strength even if constrained by injury or your physical surroundings.

Blood flow provides the oxygen and nutrients we need to perform while removing the byproducts of muscle metabolism. Get up out of your desk periodically at work to improve this process. Get up, stretch and move around and you will burn calories. It is no coincidence that people who are constantly moving tend to be thin. Conversely, people who tend to move very little are usually heavier.

If you have a sedentary job, it is essential that you get up and move around every one to two hours. It will give you a chance to breathe deeply and expand your lungs. It will give your back a break and force you to use different muscles. It aids your circulation by raising your heart rate as well as relieving the pressure on some veins that occurs while sitting.

Safety while driving is an extremely important measure of a society's and your individual health. This relates to the many effects that prolonged sitting can have on your body as well as the ability to respond to changing situations. Change positions and postures frequently while driving and take periodic breaks to keep you safe and decrease pain.

Stop every two to three hours and give your body the opportunity to improve circulation in regions that may have been compromised. Deep venous thrombosis or DVT occurs in regions that have been immobilized. Stop what you are doing and get up if you've sat in a plane or car for more than a couple hours to prevent this disastrous occurrence. Additionally, if you get up and walk around, it will relieve the pressure on your back that occurs with sitting. Get out of your car and breathe the fresh air and it will improve your wakefulness.

Muscle memory occurs in response to repetitive motions performed or postures held. These memories serve to improve postures and movements at a subconscious level. Maintain good posture at your desk will strengthen your spine while poor posture can lead to pain and fatigue. Good posture leads to increased energy and efficiency with all of your work activities.

In an ergonomic work environment, your work space is arranged in order to efficiently complete your tasks. While doing so, you while maintain good posture and use proper lift techniques. Motions done within the appropriate range of motion and with proper techniques are healthy and can improve strength. Motions done, however, with awkward postures or while overtaxing a specific joint or muscle can lead to pain and repetitive use injuries. Common repetitive use injuries include carpal tunnel syndrome and tendonitis.

Inexpensive pedometers are available that you can attach to your belt to count the steps you take throughout the day. Compare a day in which you walk the least amount possible versus a day in which you try to add extra steps. Walk instead of using your time to wait for the elevator or to find the closest parking space. You will add a significant number of steps to your day. It is remarkable how truly sedentary we can be in our society. The cumulative effect of walking more every day is improved fitness and weight maintenance.

Accessible exercise opportunities are crucial in our busy lives. There is no more accessible location than simply outside. There is no more important time to get outside than during the winter months. Absorb some sunshine during the short days and it will provide health benefits including improved bone health and elevation of mood. The boring nature of being inside all day with no good scenery can lead to seasonal affective disorders and sap your energy. The variety of activity, terrain and scenery outside creates the ideal location in which to be active.

Although not as easy as in the summer months, it is worth it to bundle up and get outside. There is no bad weather, just bad clothes. The fresh air and any sunlight you see will improve your sense of well-being and brighten your mood. Many winter sports are available as well that can get your blood pumping and challenge a competitive spirit.

In the following chapter, and you will learn how you can modify many of these everyday activities to improve something that is vital to all of us.

CHAPTER 12 - ENERGY

Efficient movement and work activities will serve to simultaneously conserve and increase your energy. Streamline and organize your environment and you will empower yourself. Avoid negative, wasteful thoughts, actions and objects and you will have the energy to truly accomplish what you want. Frustration arises when we are spinning our wheels or when obstacles block our progress.

Organize your activities with a purpose. Have a starting and stopping point and discard extraneous actions. Make a plan and stick to it. Avoid circular e-mails that decrease your efficiency and clutter your work. Pick up the phone or send a fax that provides a conclusion to the interaction. Search for purpose in your actions and interactions in your work environment and streamline when you can.

Energize your life by avoiding waste in action, diet, thought, or virtually any part of your life. The frustrations you feel are the inevitable consequences of inefficient use of your time and energy. To increase your energy, organize and streamline your life. You will feel better without the time-wasters and clutter in your life.

To save your energy at work, don't worry about what you can't control. When you can control something, however, do it. Do not spend your time on worthless e-mails. Determine which ones are relevant and act upon them. Handle paper mail only once and put it in its proper place. Keep your office organized so you do not again spend valuable time and energy searching for and reading your paperwork.

Restlessness and a feeling of unease or "stress" are the natural consequences of excessive use of computers or too much passive TV watching. Restless

Leg Syndrome, or a feeling that you want to just detach your legs and let them run around is treated primarily by increasing physical activity. Feeling tense or having an unexplained sense of urgency is undesirable energy and is our bodies' way of telling us to get up and get moving.

Activities that stimulate your mind or body will have positive consequences. A purely passive activity, like television, with no movement or interaction will leave you feeling poorly. Television has the negative effect of both not allowing your mind to relax as well as not engaging it actively. This does not apply to an educational program which holds your interest for a reasonable period of time.

If for no other reason, turn off your television and you will increase your energy level by simply giving yourself more time. If you average three hours per day of television multiplied by seven days per week, this is twenty-one hours additional time. Just think of all the ways you could use this time to improve your life. You could write a book, learn an instrument, or make the world a better place. Television does nothing to improve short or long term energy levels.

Calm energy is a feeling of being rested but also alert and aware. Television decreases your calm energy making you feel less rested and energetic and more fatigued. Worse still, watching television actually burns fifteen percent less calories than sitting still with the TV turned off.

Wakefulness is a state of being alert and consciously interactive with the environment. Light activity early in the morning can improve your energy level and alertness throughout the day. Sunlight exposure is important as well and any gentle physical activity that can de done outside provides the added benefit of helping to maintain your sleep/wake cycles. Your metabolism, or the rate at which your body burns calories, can also be jump-started by early morning activity.

Many people choose exercise first thing in the morning. This places it as a priority as it is done before any other work activities. Going forward throughout the day, you feel energized knowing that you have taken care of yourself and you may find yourself with more of an energy reserve to tackle your daily challenges.

Fatigue, or a sense of having little energy, can result from a variety of physical and emotional factors. Anxious thinking can drain your energy. Avoid worry and learn to focus your thoughts on things you can control. Be positive. Have an attitude of gratitude, and be enthusiastic. It will go a long way to increasing your energy. Fear and worry can prevent you from achieving your full potential. You will become what you think about.

Fatigue can occur from physical causes such as a lack of sleep or doing heavy physical work for an extended period of time. More often, however, it results from the thoughts that fill our heads. Worries over many things such as not having enough time or difficult relationships can drain our energy. To have the energy needed to do our best, we need to clear our minds of worry and counter-productive thinking.

Set goals and choose to excel when you compete to achieve your personal best. It will give you a measuring stick to chart your progress. Often goals are what are needed to provide the focus to keep you moving along the right path.

How you push yourself in your exercise routine is directly related to how energetic you will feel throughout the day. If you choose to compete against either your previous performances or that of others you will see and feel tangible results.

Negative energy from internal or external sources can leave us feeling drained and have a negative impact on our lives. This applies to negative energy that we direct towards others as well as thoughts and influences that we allow into our lives. Build your own firewall to protect yourself from these damaging forces.

Often our environment is filled with negativity. It may be the 24 hour news cycle or simply the attitudes of people around us. To combat these forces, seek out positive things in the world. Find a passion that refocuses your mind and renews your spirit. Spend some time to take a break and recharge your battery.

Artificial forms of energy are often substituted in our busy lives for a true, genuine and energetic life. People will try to survive on nervous, tense energy commonly fueled by caffeine. This is artificial, however, and usually precedes some degree of a collapse. Your clear thinking is harmed by the peaks and valleys that result from short term stimulation. Nervous and tense energy will keep your minds in high gear for as along as possible but, in the end, it interferes with productivity and leads to more errors. It is harder to focus or to be creative when your mind will not slow down enough to concentrate.

The natural way in which children behave when playing can be a valuable lesson for harried adults. If they feel joy they may laugh or scream. Their actions are spontaneous and unbridled. If they want to rest or to run they do so. They will listen to their bodies and, if allowed, they will do what they want and need to do. Many medical conditions such as neck and back pain, and even constipation are associated with a learned habit of denying innate cues from our bodies.

Ideamotor movement takes children naturally where they want to go. They experience joy and remain healthier by being able to move the way that they want to. Early in life, however, this begins to change as society places constraints on them and limits their freedom. Children hear "no" so many times that they lose much of their spontaneity as they mature.

Lifelong learning is another way to fill your life with energy. A sense of wonder fills you with a desire to explore new places and gives you motivation to live life to the fullest. An attitude of gratitude will help you to appreciate all that is around you. Stop to appreciate what you have been given and what you have experienced and this simple act will enrich your life. You do not want to miss it.

A sense of wonder contributes to your essential calm energy. This is energy that allows you to open your mind and truly experience the world. It is time to ponder what you're living for and why you were placed on earth. At times you need to take yourself out of gear, just coast, and enjoy the scenery around you. Learn to appreciate the simple pleasures of life and it will go a long way to energize you. It is often true that the best things in life are free. Time with friends or family costs nothing but can be priceless. Even simple smells, if you pause and allow them to register, may activate pleasure centers in your brain.

A constant search for the next best thing can leave us feeling haggard and unsatisfied. The grass is rarely greener on the other side. Energy wasted looking for something else should be directed towards what is right in front of you. The book *"A Purpose Driven Life"* demonstrates how profoundly this simple practice can change your life.

Be in tune with your mind and body and take short breaks when needed to improve your overall energy. Pause to refresh yourself and derail the build-up of stress which may occur without you being aware it is happening. Many Latin American countries take an afternoon siesta to relax and rest. Often it is done because of the heat in which they work but the result is more energy and efficiency at the end of the day.

The increased energy that comes following occasional breaks will enable you to concentrate and do more work. Bursts of energy will lead to more productivity. Your improved concentration will decrease the number of errors that you make and improve the quality of all you do.

The process of increasing your energy level can be energizing in and of itself. The way in which we travel the journey of life goes a long way to affect how we feel. Make sure you enjoy the ride and worry about the destination when you get there.

Things that we do to increase our energy level such as exercise, rest, meditation, etc. can be enjoyable and energizing unto themselves. They do not have to simply be a means to an end. Enjoy how you got there because it may be more important than where you are going. The reasons why you are pursuing your goal are often found while you are traveling towards it.

Sleep, a seemingly simple activity, has received a great deal of attention in recent years. It affects virtually every aspect of your life including your mood and energy level. Quality sleep consists of four stages that need to be passed through in order for you to awake feeling rested. Tensions or stressors that you take to bed with you will decrease the quality of your sleep and will be there when you wake up.

You need to take steps to receive the energizing benefits of sleep. Release the nervous tensions that build up throughout the day prior to going to bed and it will help you sleep. Perform activities throughout your day that benefit your energy level and they will improve your sleep. Without a release of nervous tensions, the adverse effects of poor sleep will compound with the events of the day to make you feel exhausted and drained. Quality of life is what is most positively affected by attempts to energize our lives. All aspects of work and play are affected and the time and effort it takes is truly worth it.

The net effect of seeking that which energizes you is positive both to you and others around you. They will feel your positive energy and will feel energized from it as well. Just as negativity around you can drain your energy, positive energy from within you and emitted by you to others will compound its affect. It has the power to charge your spirit.

This brings us to the concept of balance. How do you put this all together to achieve this seemingly elusive goal?

CHAPTER 13 - BALANCE

Achieve balance in your life and you have reached that midpoint where your mind and body are their most efficient. A calm sense of peace will be present in your life when is balanced properly. You can not allow one opposing force to tip the scale and pull your life in a direction that is not true to your values or priorities.

It is an elusive goal to achieve this sense of balance. To do so you have to constantly re-examine your priorities and make adjustments when necessary. The factors that unbalance your life and make it less efficient and more stressful will constantly change.

You need to filter out that which bogs you down and allow to enter your life only that which helps you keep it balanced. Periodic reexamination is needed. It may be that you need to spend more time with your spouse or children. If you are less successful or energetic than you want to be, you may need to rededicate yourself to your career or exercise program. Only by honestly taking stock of your life can you achieve the spiritual and physical balance you desire.

Participate in a variety of interesting activities to increase your chance for success. Scatter around your ideal midpoint activities that excite and energize you and ones that calm and relax you. Add fun whenever possible and it will make achieving your midpoint feel less like work

Although your midpoint may be the point at which you are most efficient, you cannot simply park in neutral and expect to be able to remain there. If a sense of peaceful restfulness is what you want to achieve, devise a thoughtful plan and execute it daily. It is an active process that requires constant rebalancing and variation of activities to maintain that point.

Dynamic (moving) and static (still) balance are critically important. Physical balance, made up of dynamic and static components, is an important aspect of the total balance we feel in our lives. At a smaller level, the multiple factors that contribute to our physical balance mirror the larger factors that contribute to an overall balanced life.

At an even smaller, local anatomic level, improved static balance results in better joint stabilization. This will help to prevent injuries and diminish the natural wear and tear on a joint. Static balance is improved through strengthening. Dynamic balance improvements occur through movement. They improve function and prevent falls and injuries

Honestly assess the progress you are making towards goals in your life. This is essential if you want to use your strengths and understanding your limitations. Listen for subtle cues that tell you that you need to make a change. Be willing to discard what is not working and try something new.

If a high energy level is your strength, you need to be in tune with any associated weakness. Avoid the limitations that may go along with being slightly hyperactive by compensating for your inevitable weaknesses. You may miss subtle meanings or not notice clues present if you do not slow down to think or to observe. Your body may tell you that you need to rest but you are not hearing it. Hyperkinetic activity can damage interpersonal relationships if you do not slow down to listen or to respect others feelings. Conversely, being too sedentary or overly pensive can be a negative drag on those around you.

The uniqueness of your skill set and abilities will affect how we perform. If speed is your forte, you will gravitate towards exercises in which you can use your speed to excel. The success you achieve will make exercise more enjoyable. In sports, you will naturally assume positions in which quickness is essential. Strength may be the defining factor for another athlete. He or she may not be the fastest but they can use their strength to succeed in the gym and on the field. For others, finesse may be their strong point. They may be very smooth and efficient with their movements and be considered a "cerebral" athlete.

Athletes who can combine and balance all of these factors are able to achieve great power. Institutes dedicated to improving speed and strength enable athletes to create more power and do more work. They run programs that vary the exercise routine and improve both speed and strength

A universal truth in all exercise programs is that you must do some form of resistance or strengthening exercises. To achieve peak performance, your muscles will need to be strong. They will respond to stresses placed upon them. To get them to improve you will need to occasionally push them to the point of fatigue to cause subtle breakdown. Your body will then respond by building your up muscles.

Moderate muscle soreness the day following strenuous exercise lets you know that you are pushing your muscles hard enough. This results from micro- tearing of muscle fibers as well as build up of byproducts of metabolism such as lactic acid. Strength balanced with the right amount of speed and flexibility will lead to maximum performance and less injuries.

Motivation to continue exercise comes from small successes which you realize. Set realistic goals and it will help keep you headed in the right direction. Balanced goals result in balanced outcomes. Achievements you make along the way serve as benchmarks of progress towards your goals.

Without goals, you may be drift aimlessly. Goals provide the subtle motivation you need to continue. Goals can be short or long term. A short term goal may be to simply get to the gym three times a week. A long term goal may be to lower your body fat by 5% or your cholesterol by twenty points. Take stock of where we are at, where we want to be and how to get there with measurable goals.

Rebounding from a disturbance defines resilience. People with great resilience have a unique ability to maintain or regain normal function and balance following an injury or a stress. Nurture your capacity to return to a consistent level of structure and function and it will help you achieve peak functioning over the long run.

At the cellular level, resilience manifests itself as the power of a cell to recover back to its original shape and size after removal of the strain which caused the deformation. On a larger scale, this is represented functionally by "muscle memory." This results in the ability of a muscle to move in known patterns, improve performance and make activities feel more natural. Following injury, a system with better developed muscle memory will recover its form and function more quickly.

Efficient, balanced use of your whole system enables you to sustain a prolonged stressful effort. Stamina is the ability to sustain this balanced endurance and vigor. A high degree of stamina is essential to consistently perform at a high level throughout a competition.

Have stamina and you have the physical strength to resist or withstand fatigue and hardship. This difference can determine a champion. Stamina is a key ingredient of a competition like the Tour de France. Without a doubt, Lance Armstrong had enduring physical and mental energy and strength that allowed him to compete for an extended period of time. The principal foundation or backbone of all sustained activities is our stamina.

Draw your muscles out to their full length and it will enable them to function throughout their full range of motion. This will lead to balanced function throughout a larger range. Stretch your muscles and tendons and it will extend their length and breadth and help you to avoid injury and improve your performance.

Extend a muscle beyond its ordinary limit in a controlled fashion and it will increase performance, speed recovery and avoid injury. As you stretch your muscles you may also be able to extend the scope of what you have been capable of doing. You can "stretch the limits" of your running, jumping, lifting, etc. Reach out and stretch beyond your usual limits and it will extend your horizon and broaden your performance range.

Smart snacking is essential to balance your energy levels and fuel your activities. Snacking is often associated with an unhealthy diet because of the easy availability of unhealthy choices. When used correctly, snacking is an important component of a healthy diet. The key is to keep snacking in perspective and pay attention to what you eat. Provide yourself optimum benefit by properly timing what you eat.

Advance preparation is the secret to healthy snacking. Healthy snacks can provide the fiber and nutrients your body needs. Take the time to prepare homemade snacks because they are the healthiest. You control the ingredients as well as the size of the portion. These may include fruit, dry vegetables, yogurt or endless other natural options. When this is not possible, look for small portion snacks like the new 100 calorie snack packs. They primarily address portion size which is one of the biggest diet-wrecking culprits. Read the label and avoid trans-fat or excessive simple carbohydrates.

Tone, the continuous, partial contraction of muscles is another essential component of balance. If a sudden stretch occurs or a disruption of your equilibrium occurs, the body maintains balance by reflexively increasing the muscle's tension. The ability to do this improves your athletic performance and guards you against injury or danger. Further, muscle tone improves your appearance and supports your posture.

Unconscious nerve impulses maintain the passive, continuous partial contractions that maintain balance and support the framework of who we are. Although there is an underlying, subconscious steady-state contraction of the muscles in your body, there is much you can do to affect muscle tone and posture. In general, the adage of 'strengthen what's weak and stretch what's tight' holds true. Work on high repetition exercises to emphasize muscle tone over bulk. Back extension exercises help to maintain an upright posture. These active, conscious exercises improve tone and provide subconscious postural strength and pain relieving benefits throughout the day.

Transitions provide connections between all the aspects of your exercise program. A transition such as a cool-down period is the time to tune in to and react to unique feedback from your body. Time your transitions from warm-up to strenuous exercise and back to a cool-down period in an organized and balanced manner.

The warm-up period, includes stretching followed by a gradual increase in the strenuousness of your exercise. It improves range of motion, reduces risk of injury, decreases post-exercise muscle pain and delayed-onset muscle soreness. Transition to a cool-down period with gentle active and passive stretching and a gradual reduction in intensity of activity to complete a balanced training regimen.

Alternate brief periods of increased speed and exertion with sustained exercise in your workout. This is the basis of interval training. To achieve strength and conditioning gains, insert periods of high intensity work into your regimen. By doing so, you can prevent an over-training effect that can occur with doing the same thing repetitively.

Your body will adapt to interval training in ways that will help improve your conditioning and performance. New blood vessels will form that improves the circulation to your muscles. You will improve the transportation of oxygen to your muscles as well as the transportation of waste products such as lactate away from your muscles. In doing so, you achieve both an aerobic and anaerobic benefit. You will be better able to use stored energy and oxygen during periods of high intensity work for a sustained level of aerobic activity.

Increase power and speed by adding bursts to your exercise routine. Similar to interval training, they consist of brief periods of explosive movement. They can improve sports performance and provide gains in speed and strength and add balance to your training regimen.

More sophisticated burst or interval training regimens are specifically tailored to a sports-specific activity. Sports medicine specialists or trainers can evaluate the activity and mimic it in your training program. A running back, for example, should balance brief, intense activities requiring maximum strength and acceleration with periods of sustained exertion. For the casual athlete, bursts provide the added benefit of increasing your metabolism after your workout is completed which burns more calories and fat throughout the day.

In the following chapter, you will learn how exercise can be viewed as a prescription.

CHAPTER 14 - EXERCISE AS A PRESCRIPTION

As pharmaceutical prices have risen, it has become good medicine to view exercise as a prescription. It is a safe, widely available, and economical option to improve health and combat disease. In most cases, it is free. Virtually anyone can safely exercise. An exercise program should begin with a physician's prescription listing relevant diagnoses, which activities to perform, and which ones to avoid.

More specifically, your physician should list your diagnosis (if applicable), the specific type of exercise, frequency and duration. He or she will consider your overall health, interests and goals to make your experience both safe and productive. It is also an opportunity to discuss the expectations of your exercise program as well as any contraindications that may exist such as previous injuries or medical conditions.

A doctor may prescribe exercise for weight loss because of its ability to both suppress your appetite and burn calories. Because of this, exercise is the most effective way to achieve ideal weight. Walk at a leisurely pace and you will burn approximately 250 calories/hour. More brisk walking can burn 400 calories/hour. Combine this with the fact that exercise can take away your appetite for sixty to eighty minutes following an intense activity and it is easy to see how weight loss occurs.

Following intense exercise, you will continue to burn more calories because of an increased metabolic rate and blood flow. You will further avoid many of the emotional cues that lead to overeating i.e. T.V. or boredom. Beware the practice of overcompensating for the amount of calories you think you have burnt. Sugar-laden sports drinks are notorious culprits. It is easy to cancel the weight loss benefits of exercise if you reward yourself consistently with food.

Add muscle as another way to increase the number of calories you burn. For every extra pound of muscle added, your body burns an extra fifty calories per day. Regular weight training can boost your metabolic rate significantly. This is because your muscle is more vascular, does more work and is more metabolically active. Your muscle will continue to work for you, even at rest, to burn more calories.

To build muscle you need to move and, by doing so, you will burn more calories. Active people who move throughout the day can burn twice as many calories as more sedentary individuals. Weight training keeps you strong and active as you age, and enables you to continue to perform cardiovascular exercises and to enjoy your avocational activities.

Include high intensity exercise in your workout to most effectively burn fat. The exercise prescription for fat burning includes periods of intense exercise added to sustained lighter exercise. A method of doing this is to sprint or pedal rapidly "spinning" for short bursts on a stationary bike.

Bursts of higher intensity followed by a period of recovery will further allow you to achieve greater heart rate variability. This is the difference between your resting and maximum heart rate and a great predictor of health. The burst of activity will also sustain an elevated heart rate for up to an hour, a period commonly called the "afterburn." The ultimate goal is fitness, but to burn those extra fat calories and lose weight, it is essential to add bursts of higher intensity.

Your physician's prescription may stress weight maintenance after hitting your target weight. Weight stability is the ultimate goal. If you have dieted for a period of time, you are going to want to resume more normal eating habits. To avoid an unhealthy yo-yo effect of weight loss and gain you need to increase your calorie intake slowly. Start first with larger portions of healthy foods rather than adding junk food. Weigh yourself once a week. If your weight is staying stable, you've hit the right mark.

Ultimately, the key is to maintain a healthy weight through an active lifestyle. If after the first week you have noticed any weight gain, you either must cut back on the food or increase your activity. This applies to you only if your primary goal is weight loss and not to build muscle. To lose one pound, you must burn 3,500 calories more than you have consumed. This works out to 500 calories per day for a whole week. Knowing this, it is easy to see how excess calories can really add up.

Exercise as a prescription for cardiovascular and pulmonary health can also reap great rewards. Aerobic exercises that require increased oxygen consumption for a sustained period of time are often prescribed. For people with pulmonary disease, specific exercises can be done such as pursed-lip breathing or rib expansion exercises to improve the body's ability to obtain oxygen and exchange carbon dioxide.

The benefits of aerobic exercises extend throughout the body. They will lead to a lower resting heart rate as your body becomes more efficient. You will also increase your ability to raise your heart rate and do more work. Aerobic exercises can also prevent the cardiopulmonary deconditioning that can lead to debility. Once you start these healthy practices, however, you should never stop as the benefits can be quickly lost.

Fitness and exercise can extend your life and improve its quality and allow you to be more active and productive. It will make life more pleasant and enjoyable as you age. Further, remain strong and fit and it will improve your balance and prevent falls when you become elderly. From a mental health standpoint, the socialization that comes with exercise participation will elevate your mood and keep your mind sharp.

Many people think that as we age, physical decline is an inevitable part of the process. In large measure, this is not true. Most of the physical frailty associated with advanced age is the result of inactivity. By improving your lifestyle, this can be significantly improved. Physical activity also protects against other chronic diseases such as heart disease, osteoporosis, diabetes and depression.

Osteoporosis is a condition in which your bones have a decreased bone mineral density. This makes them more fragile and easier to break. These osteoporotic fractures can lead to catastrophic consequences in the elderly. Many new pills to treat this condition have come on the market in the last few years but none are more effective than exercise. Because bones are dynamic structures, exercise can improve bone strength as bones react to forces applied across them. Jogging, walking or stair climbing at 70-90% of maximum effort three times per week, along with 1500 mg of calcium per day can increase bone density of the lower spine by 5% in nine months.

Good posture contributes both as a cause and effect of osteoporosis. Good posture cannot prevent osteoporosis but it may decrease its effects. Consciously stand up straight to maintain the back extensor muscle strength that is essential for good posture. Vertebral fractures of the spine, seen in people with osteoporosis, will lead to poor posture, compromise respiration, and adversely effect mobility. Exercises can improve your posture even if this has occurred and improve your strength and balance.

Doctors may also prescribe exercise to improve bowel and bladder function. Transit time through your alimentary canal is significantly accelerated by moderate exercise. Inactivity reduces bowel function but exercise helps stimulate the bowels. Remain adequately hydrated while exercising in order for this to work correctly.

Kegel exercises are often prescribed to improve urinary incontinence. Strengthen the muscles of the pelvic floor by consciously contracting and relaxing these muscles to decrease urinary incontinence and minimize the effects of uterine prolapse. To do this, contract the muscles that you would use to stop urinating and hold it for a few seconds. Do this several times a day to strengthen your pelvic muscles and improve both bowel and bladder control.

Improve your lab values such as cholesterol and blood glucose with regular aerobic exercise. The positive feedback that you get when your lab values are reviewed will motivate you to continue to exercise. You can avoid the side effects of medications and raise your HDL or good cholesterol, and lower the LDL, or bad cholesterol. Exercise will also improve your circulation and increase your body's ability to clear away clots in blood vessels.

Exercise decreases insulin resistance and improves your body's ability to handle glucose. Exercise and weight loss are the initial treatment prescriptions for type II diabetics. It improves their insulin resistance and may normalize blood glucose. As glycemic control improves, there initially is a need for close monitoring of blood sugars and fluid intake. In the long run, however, exercise can lead to fewer type II diabetics and less of a need for glucose monitoring.

Mood and affect can also be treated with exercise. Exercise effects brain chemistry in ways that are similar to the mechanism of commonly prescribed antidepressants. Blood levels of serotonin and endorphins are increased in people who regularly perform aerobic exercise. Regular exercise can allow some people to taper off their antidepressants. Exercise is an easy, inexpensive way to improve mood and better deal with stress.

You can improve your overall sense of well-being through chemical changes that occur. Serotonin levels in the brain are a key component of mood. Its levels are increased with exercise. Anyone who runs long distances can describe the feeling of the runners high. It has been linked to chemicals called endorphins. These chemicals were found to be similar to morphine in chemical structure and pain killing ability. By improving your sense of well-being, you can better block out irrelevant stressors. Your improved overall condition gives you the endurance you need to complete longer tasks. Exercise, however, must be done on a regular basis to maintain its positive benefits.

Improve mental performance measures by exercise. It positively affects alertness, focus and concentration. It provides a time during physical exertion when you can mentally process ideas and make plans for action once you get back to work. After exercise, people are better able to concentrate and act upon information. It improves the ability to block out irrelevant information.

Further, exercise improves your speed of decision making. Multiple variables affect overall cognition function. These include your ability to sustain attention to the task, remember what you need to remember and process the information. Exercise releases chemicals that are beneficial to the brain's processing system. It has also been shown to increase the number of neuronal connections in the brain which improves cognitive function and prevents cognitive decline late in life.

Improve your capacity for self-healing, or your body's innate ability to restore balance and function by exercising regularly. Many of the benefits of exercise extend to the body's ability to heal itself. Shorten your convalescent period following injury through gentle exercise. Strength, circulation and oxygenation are improved. These aid healing and assist the body in the delivery of nutrients and removal of waste products.

Exercise helps to boost the immune system and regulate the hormones that influence healing. At the same time, you receive the obvious benefits of improved strength and endurance. Prevent much of the stiffness and weakness that would occur by continuing to exercise appropriately while recovering from an injury. Minimize the loss of muscle memory and you can return to maximum performance more quickly.

Target sore or injured areas with exercise and therapy as soon as possible. Manual therapies consisting of gentle tissue mobilization, modalities such as heat or ice, and stretching or strengthening exercises can be specifically directed at an injured area. At times, however, it is appropriate to completely rest an injured area. If there is any doubt, ask your doctor. An example may be a severely injured upper extremity that needs to be immobilized. In this case, focus your exercises on your lower body to avoid generalized deconditioning. As soon as it is appropriate, however, you should begin to exercise the injured area.

Under the direction of your physician, you may initially begin resistance-free range of motion exercises or isometric exercises with no joint movement. It is important for recovery as well as future injury prevention to begin to strengthen the injured region and supporting structures. Typically, the more mild the injury, the sooner exercise should begin. When it comes to low back pain, an early and consistent exercise program is the single most important factor for both short and long term prognosis.

Exercise is also prescribed for cosmetic reasons. Your appearance is determined in part by factors such as body shape, muscle tone and skin. Exercise will improve all of these aspects. Exercise will increase your muscle mass and decrease your body fat. This in conjunction with the genetic framework you were born with will determine your shape. Exercise improves your posture, and maximizes your ability to project strength and confidence.

Motivate yourself to start exercising and to continue exercising in whatever way you like. Appearance is a legitimate motivator even though the health benefits are the most important factors. Trying to look like a model on a cover of a magazine may be an elusive goal but it still may keep you moving in the right direction.

In the next chapter, I'll discuss a treatment philosophy that improves health, performance and decreases pain.

CHAPTER 15 - OSTEOPATHIC MANIPULATION

Osteopathic manipulation consists of manual therapy to diagnose, treat and prevent illness or disease. Osteopathic physicians or D.O.'s use their hands to improve blood and lymphatic flow, balance movement, and restore function in their patients. By studying the relationship between structure and function, D.O.'s can improve athletic performance and speed healing.

The osteopathic physician's role is to find alterations in structure and, by using manipulation, improve their function. A patient may complain of chronic hip pain, for example, while exercising. By examining the overall structure, the doctor may discover a distant alteration that could be manually corrected. This would improve their gait and decrease their pain.

At the core of the osteopathic philosophy is a belief in the body's innate ability to heal itself. A.T. Still, the founder of Osteopathy, said, "The rule of the artery is supreme." This means that good circulation is essential to relieve tissue congestion and remove toxins. Correct musculoskeletal functioning is essential to ensure good circulation and to facilitate healing.

By improving the body's structure and function, it is better able to maintain health. For the athlete or those in exercise programs, this is invaluable to limit the effects of nagging injuries. Osteopathic manipulation focuses on the whole body, while emphasizing soft tissue, neuromuscular and skeletal structures. It is effective to improve healing and prevent injury.

Somatic dysfunction is defined as an "impaired or altered function of related components of the somatic (body framework) system: skeletal, arthrodial and myofascial structures and related vascular, lymphatic and neural elements." In short, somatic dysfunction is where we direct our care.

Just as important as the somatic components are the related vascular, lymphatic and neural elements. Rarely, does a problem exist in isolation. The Osteopathic Physician examines the chief complaint and devises a treatment plan as it affects the related elements. The elements are interrelated and as the somatic system improves so will its related elements. Conversely, improvements in circulation and the neurological system will improve the musculoskeletal function and recovery.

TART is an acronym for what Osteopathic Physicians diagnose when they examine a dysfunctional or painful area. It stands for tissue texture changes, asymmetry, range of motion and tenderness. Tissue texture changes are what an experienced examiner feels when he or she is palpating soft tissue. Asymmetry corresponds to side to side differences in multiple physical factors. Range of motion is tested both actively and passively. Tenderness is usually the subjective complaint that brings the patient to our office.

Using osteopathic manipulation, we approach the components of somatic dysfunction in combination. Often, what we do to treat one area takes care of multiple other ones. Manual therapy that improves range of motion frequently will decrease pain. The Osteopathic Physician will usually treat areas of concern as they are discovered as opposed to planning on coming back to them. This provides benefits that build upon themselves.

Barriers are an important concept in manual medicine. Barriers provide the end-range of active or passive range of motion. They can be anatomic, meaning that they are the end-range of motion based on solid anatomic structures. They can be elastic, indicating there is no hard end range but rather an area of increasing resistance based upon stretch. Physiologic barriers mark the expected, natural range of motion.

Manual medicine is directed at restrictive or pathologic barriers. These exist due to injury or imbalances. Manual medicine addresses these barriers in a direct or indirect manner. To treat directly, the physician goes directly up against the restrictive barriers and then tries to move directly through it to restore more normal range of motion. To treat indirectly, the physician moves away from the barrier attempting to reset balance and restore a more normal range of motion.

A.T. Still was an Allopathic physician who founded Osteopathic Medicine after the Civil War. He witnessed the death of several of his children and he felt that there had to be a better way to care for sick people. At that time, medications were often ineffective. From his grief, he ultimately created a system of healthcare that relied more on the body's innate ability to heal itself and less on the medications that were available at that time.

Over the years there has been a significant convergence in the osteopathic and allopathic medical professions. Many Allopathic Physicians have received additional training in manual medicine and some Osteopathic physicians don't use the manual the skills that they were taught in medical school. Additionally, the majority of osteopathic medical students currently complete an allopathic residency. The challenge is to continue to combine the manual and structural skills within an excellent medical system.

When a physician takes a holistic approach to the treatment of the patient it means they treat the whole body. There is always a risk of looking at a problem in isolation and not putting it in its proper context of the whole person. Homeostasis is achieved when all the components of the body are in balance and this is what we seek to achieve. Osteopathic manipulation requires us to look at the patient with a broad vision.

By taking a more holistic approach, you can more successfully treat multiple confounding factors that are worsening the chief complaint. Somatic or musculoskeletal reflections of internal problems are frequently found. These are painful soft tissue changes palpated by the physician. When treated, they improve the visceral ailment. In addition, diet, sleep, exercise and lifestyle in general are all examined when treating a patient holistically.

Manual therapy today is performed by a variety of practitioners. In many instances, the procedures are similar to those done by an Osteopathic Physician. Manual therapy has never been the property of one specialty. The osteopathic profession from its inception has sought to educate multiple disciplines including chiropractic, physical therapy and neuromuscular therapy.

Chiropractors frequently use direct force to correct vertebral subluxations. They do this with direct hands-on adjustments or through the use of mechanical devices. Many physical therapists have begun to do soft tissue myofascial release in conjunction with exercise to maximize their outcome. This is a gentler form of manual therapy that compliments their exercise program. Neuromuscular therapists perform manual therapy consisting of deep soft tissue massage, trigger point release or perpendicular massage to relieve spasm and decrease pain.

Direct manipulation techniques involve moving to and then through a barrier. A direct manipulation technique called high velocity low amplitude or HVLA manipulation involves engaging a barrier and then rapidly moving through it with a brief thrust. This technique is what most people associate with an "adjustment" and may result in a cracking or popping sound. This sound is not essential, however, for the adjustment to have been effective.

Mobilization with impulse is another way to describe high velocity manipulation. A brief impulse is provided by the physician to provide mobilization of the restricted segment. Once a direct release is done to an area of somatic dysfunction, it is often easier and more effective to perform soft tissue or other indirect techniques. Following this, the patient is educated on what exercises they should do to maintain balance and prevent recurrence.

Counterstrain is a theory of osteopathic manipulation that works by directing attention to the strain reflex. The osteopathic Physician identifies the somatic dysfunction as tenderness, tissue texture changes or abnormal range of motion. To treat, he seeks a position of ease at which the pain level of the trigger point is decreased by at least 50%. He does this by passively moving the patient's body into a position in which a release is felt below his finger and the patient reports 50% pain relief. This position is then held for 90 seconds.

Modifications of Counterstrain include Still Release Techniques and Facilitated Positional Release. Still Release Techniques, as devised by Dr. Richard VanBuskirk involve finding the position of ease as is done with counterstrain. He positions the appropriate part of the axial or appendicular spine, applies a compressive or distractive force and then takes it through a range of motion. He based his treatment model on old black and white footage of A.T. Still himself treating a patient. Facilitated positional release is a time efficient modification of counterstrain devised by Dr. Stanley Schiowitz. He finds the position of ease and then provides a distraction or compression force to rapidly treat each area and save the 60-90 seconds that it takes to treat each point.

Palpatory feedback is an essential component of myofascial release. It is a skill learned mastered by constantly being in tune to the information coming in through your fingers. Lightly feeling the soft tissues gives the examiner a great deal of information. The doctor uses the palpatory information to treat the painful area in a direct or indirect manner.

Trigger points by their nature refer or trigger pain to a different part of the body. Classic referral patterns have been mapped out over the years and give diagnostic clues to the responsible part of the body. To treat these points directly, the physician gently guides the soft tissue up against the barrier waiting for the "creep" or release to occur. In an indirect manner, the physician moves the soft tissue away from the barrier in order to achieve a release or new balance.

Muscle energy or "contract and relax" is a form of Osteopathic Manipulation intended to increase range of motion and improve function. The Physician or Therapist passively takes the joint to the end of its range of motion. The patient then contracts his muscles against the physician's hands to prevent joint movement. As the patient relaxes, the physician simultaneously takes up the slack and gently increases the range of motion.

Stretching is often impeded by inadequate relaxation or by the firing of the muscle stretch reflex. Muscle energy can prevent both of these from occurring when they are done correctly. You can also do it independently without the assistance of a physician or therapist. To perform it on your neck, for example, rotate it to one side, contract gently against your hand, relax, and then guide your neck a few degrees further.

Physical therapy and therapeutic exercises are important extensions of osteopathic manipulation. Manipulation assists with pain relief and improves mobility and allows physical therapy to be more effective. A good therapist identifies barriers and corrects them by a form of manual release. They may identify areas of hyper or hypo mobility that can be specifically treated. The correct balance of strength and flexibility maintains the benefits achieved through manual therapy.

Once the areas of somatic dysfunction are corrected, the body will respond better to exercise. It will then be able to function at its highest level. Exercise will also help to maintain the strength and functional gains that have been achieved. Without strengthening, the body may quickly revert back to its painful, dysfunctional pattern. It is therefore essential that you be an active participant in your care. The manual correction is only the beginning

Ideally, manipulation should be done on an episodic, time limited basis. The Mercy Consensus Guidelines for Chiropractic Manipulation warn that excessive manipulation can lead to a dependence on passive care and an over reliance on physician intervention. My goal is to transition the patient to active, self-directed care as soon as it is possible. This includes a multitude of things including strengthening and stretching as well as self application of modalities such as heat or ice.

As an adjunct to active treatment, manual therapy is invaluable. It helps you improve your body awareness and achieve optimal function. It may release areas of somatic dysfunction that you did not know existed which were causing pain or restricting movement. Ultimately, your health can improve with appropriate use of manipulation.

In the next chapter, you will learn how proper focus throughout life will increase your success

CHAPTER 16 - FOCUS

Focus your exercise program on your goals and balance your approach to maximize your performance. Exercise all sections of your body equally to achieve physical balance. Strengthen your body in a symmetrical manner with equal attention to anterior, posterior and side to side musculature. In a broader sense, balance relates to all aspects of your life. For optimal health and well-being, focus on balancing all the areas that contribute to your personal quality of life.

Nowhere is there more attention paid to the concepts of focus and balance than the martial arts disciplines. They train their students to focus their minds and bodies to achieve optimal strength and balance. They may not carry the most muscle bulk or be the fastest runner but their overall performance level is second to none.

Consistent, focused, life-long exercise is what is needed to achieve the maximum health benefits. In order to do this, you must vary your activities over time. People that are effective at this balance many different activities over the years. Retired, competitive football players, for example, realize that the intense strengthening or explosive exercises they did when they were young are no longer appropriate after they have stopped playing. For these large statured athletes to remain healthy, primarily aerobic exercises with only light weight training is ideal.

To prevent the detrimental health effects of being out in poor physical condition, continue to exercise throughout your life. You lose it in far less time than it takes to gain it back. It's not even close. To prevent this, vary your activities and adapt as needed to prevent burnout and overuse injuries.

Vary your routine and participate in a variety of activities and you will see a positive impact. Children who participate in a variety of different sports while growing up will in general be the healthiest, most well-rounded adults. This is counter to the current trend to deemphasize physical education or condense it to brief four to six week periods, like "summer gym". We need to teach them to be active every day. The NFL has begun to speak out on the need for regular physical activity with their Play 60 campaign. They encourage children to be physically active at least 60 minutes a day. Some video game consoles will even pause and encourage children to go outside and play!

To decrease the wear and tear on specific joints, perform multiple different activities throughout your week. If you are a regular runner, it is wise to occasionally decrease the number of miles you run and do more low impact aerobics such as biking or swimming. Focus on a variety of activities to strengthen muscles that support more vulnerable regions such as the knees or low back. This further decreases the wear and tear when you return to your regular activity.

Fit, elderly people are a testament to the effect of remaining active and the importance of varying your activities. Jack Lalane, born in 1914, often called the Godfather of Fitness looks like he is in his fifties even though he is 95 years old. As a young child, he ate an unhealthy diet of junk food and sugar. At age 15 because of the way he felt, he decided to change his life and exercise and eat a healthy diet. He has a singular focus that has motivated him throughout his life. The rest, you could say, is history.

As a young man, he entered chiropractor school but soon left to open his own gym. He initially emphasized weight lifting for both men and women and then diversified his philosophies over the years. He advocated swimming and became an accomplished swimmer late in life. He actually swam the English Channel pulling a tug boat. He included many aerobic exercises in his long running TV program as well as his tapes, books and presentations. He's educated many people on healthy eating. His famous juicer allows an easy way to drink fruits and vegetables while saving the fiber for other baking needs.

Like no other sport, baseball demonstrates how older athletes can continue to excel if they focus on excellence. Pitchers, like Roger Clemens, recorded some of their greatest performances after age 40. Alleged steroid use notwithstanding, he did so by working hard at his exercise routine and being a fierce competitor.

Rather than simply throwing all the time, high level pitchers sustain their careers by varying their exercise routine and strengthening their base of support. Roger Clemens was famous for focusing on his gluteal muscles which function as hip extensors and abductors. When these muscles are stronger, there is more push-off available there is to be transferred up to the arms.

The ability to take your performance to the next higher level is the ultimate goal of many elite athletes. Once a high level of performance has been achieved, breaking through is often the most difficult step. Michael Jordan was famous for the grueling workouts that he went through during the second Chicago Bulls "3-peat." Even though he was arguably the best basketball player to have ever played the game, he never lost the passion to succeed. His focus drove him elevate his game to the highest level and to continued success late in his basketball career.

Continuous Performance Improvement (CPI) is a dynamic process used to improve all aspects of business. It is called Karzin by the Japanese and was first implemented after World War II. High level athletes functioning on teams are synonymous in many ways to members of a business. In this model, the head coaches are the CEOs. To be effective the coaches and athletes must think systematically while considering both the process and its results while continuously reexamining the assumptions that are driving behavior.

Love what you do and find your passion and it will go a long way to inspire and motivate you to continue. Bob Feller, even though he's greater than 90years old, still works at fantasy baseball camps. He obviously loves baseball and this has kept him active and healthy. He is able to make his work fun and he continues to inspire others.

Find a form of exercise that you enjoy and focus on what makes you happy and improves your life. You must always look for what will inspire you to improve and stay the course that leads you to this goal. For some people, training for periodic competition like 5K races, gives them a goal to focus their attention. For others, it may be group exercise that inspires them because of the socialization it provides.

Maintain a young attitude by playing games throughout your life. Play can transform many mundane activities, including exercise or daily chores, into fun. In the past, constructive play prevented much of the obesity that we see currently. Today, we can complete many of our tasks and participate in modern leisure activities without ever leaving our chair. To combat this, find what you enjoy and do it on a regular basis. Play is a large part of a happy and healthy life. Even if your tasks feel like drudgery, modify them in a way to make them enjoyable. It can be sometimes done with the simplest of acts.

Modify your actions and seek continuous quality improvement to achieve above and beyond your expected physical capacities. Many famous athletes overachieved by focusing on specific talents and using this knowledge to change their routine. Michael Irvin, for example, excelled by being, as Troy Aikman put it, "the strongest person at the point of the catch". He used a burst of strength at the moment of the catch and this greatly increased his effectiveness. Barry Sanders mastered an uncanny ability to change direction and elude runners. At his Hall of Fame acceptance speech he made the comment that if he could survive working on hot roofs with his dad, then playing football would be easy. Bernie Kosar became one of the greatest quarterbacks in Cleveland Browns history by relying on his intelligence and accuracy.

A common thread that runs through all of these athletes was a love of what they were doing. They took what others would consider work and incorporated it into what they loved in their lives. In order to continue doing what they loved they continuously focused on their strengths and ultimately achieved great success.

Benefits of games and exercises are felt in many ways throughout the day. For those who exercise or compete in a sport at the end of the day, the simple anticipation of the activity can be a motivating factor. It will make it easier to focus on your work and make your day go by a little more smoothly. If you exercise early in the morning, you will have an improved sense of calm and wakefulness throughout the day. Your alertness, focus, and energy are increased by elevating your heart rate and getting your blood pumping early in the morning. Internally, your body will transition more efficiently from the sleep hormone melatonin to the mood elevating hormone serotonin.

Exercise to improve your mood while becoming physically fit. Mood improvement includes both stress reduction, mood elevation and an increased sense of calm. In Physical Medicine, exercise is a cornerstone of our treatment plans. For chronic pain patients, mood disturbances are frequently present. Even if their pain does not change, exercise improves their ability to cope with their pain, function at a higher level, and focus on other aspects of their life. Because of its profound effects, Jack Lalane has said, "Exercise is king and diet is queen and together they make a dynasty."

In the movie City Slickers, the character played by Jack Palance told the city dwellers that they all had to find "the one thing." Once they found it, they would know that that was what they should focus upon. They looked at him curiously and were initially frustrated. By the end of the movie, they knew what he meant. It was whatever inspired them or gave them purpose.

When it comes to exercise, the "one thing" may be the simplest action that enables you to stick with your routine it and continue your program. A home gym works best for some people. Maximize your chance for success with a sense of ownership of the equipment and the familiar environment of your home. I encourage older people to work in their garden or yard as another great way to stay healthy. Improved fitness will be the natural side effect of the gardening they accomplish. For other people, a dedicated club for running, biking or hiking may provide the one thing that is needed to sustain their interest in these activities.

Immediate and long term benefits come from regular exercise. Strength will improve and your endurance will increase. This will enable you to do your work more safely and with greater efficiency. Your energy levels will improve and make you less susceptible to sickness. Exercise also puts force across your bones that help to keep them strong and resistant to fractures.

Initially, you will see rapid changes in strength and speed. Over the Long run, this high rate of improvement does not continue but what does happen is that lifelong health benefits are realized. This includes everything from a reduction in cardiovascular risk factors to an improvement in health of your skin.

Time management has been referred to a practice that allows individuals to make the best use of their time. Blend activities and focus on more than one task at once and it will allow you to simultaneously complete more than one goal. If you are a multi-tasking, Type A person, daily exercise just for the sake of exercise may be monotonous. Add an activity such as coaching and it will fulfill your desire to exercise while accomplishing something else. You can focus on teaching, demonstrate sports activities, and realize health benefits for yourself all at the same time.

For others, exercise can occur while practicing with your children. You will see the added benefit of improved skill and confidence in your children and the benefit of exercise in yourself. Ultimately, you cannot save or even manage time. All you can do is spend your time. Spend your time wisely and manage your daily activities and accomplish tasks in a healthy way.

There are abundant avenues that allow virtually everybody to compete and lead a healthy lifestyle. The National Senior Games Association is a prime example. It is dedicated to motivating senior men and women to focus on a healthy lifestyle. It further supports education and research to promote ways of ensuring healthy aging. The closely related Senior Olympics began as a program theme called "Lifetime Sports." This theme, begun in the 1960's by the National Recreation Association, supported the concept that emphasis should be placed on getting individuals involved in sports in which they could compete throughout their lifespan.

The Special Olympics and programs sponsored by the MDA are two other examples of opportunities that allow everyone to compete. In both cases, activities and equipment are modified to allow the participants to compete on a level playing field. No matter your age or unique situation, opportunities to participate are available.

Leisure, a period of time spent out of work, is an important aspect of our lives. Leisure activities consist of the choices we make regarding what to do with our free time. Loosely defined, it is the period of time before and after things that we must do.

Although leisure can mean many different things, it universally represents freedom from time-consuming activities. It provides an opportunity to focus on something of your own choice. It may be exactly the same as a work activity, but done within the confines of free choice, it represents something much different. A correct balance between leisure and work needs to be found and it is different for everyone. To lead a healthy life, you need to have time at your own command that is free from compulsory engagement.

In the following chapter, I discuss how different exercise philosophies can guide your exercise routines.

CHAPTER 17 – PHILOSOPHIES OF EXERCISE

Philosophies of exercise vary widely. They approach the goal of optimal health and performance from different angles but the outcome can be quite similar. Exercise philosophies vary greatly and range from the ancient martial arts to modern programs such as Pilates.

Control is a hallmark of the martial arts. Practitioners learn to discipline both their emotions and actions. The respect that is engrained in the minds of martial arts students translates to a program that encompasses both fitness and self defense. It simultaneously empowers them while at the same time teaching humility. Manners and code of conduct are essential. Their philosophies can transcend the fighting ring and extend to every day experiences in which balance and control are needed.

Karate teaches you to channel energy and use it to maximize the effectiveness and efficiency of natural movements. Karate literally means "empty hands." At its core, it emphasizes the power of the individual and the positive energy that exists inside them to provide self defense and move in the right direction.

The base of support from which your power originates is the key to the success of karate. No weapons are used besides the individual's own power to provide self-defense. The combatant creates natural but powerful movements as the energy flows from within him.

Tao Bo is a relatively new variation of martial arts that adds a significant component of aerobics. It borrows many of the kicks and punches from karate and adds them to an aerobic program to create a more comprehensive exercise routine. It emphasizes both fitness and strength.

It makes exercise more enjoyable as it adds rhythmic dance moves to the exercise routine.

Use good technique to avoid injuries while training and exercising and this will help you to prevent injuries while playing your sport. In athletics, you want your exercise routine to improve your performance. You must be careful, however, to make sure that your routine is not having detrimental long term effects on your body. Tae Bo is an exercise routine that fulfills this mandate. Because it is low impact, it avoids the forceful pounding on your joints. It improves strength and emphasizes stretching which increases the safe range of motion of your joints.

Pilates is a popular philosophy of exercise that was created by Joseph Pilates during the First World War. Pilates developed "The Pilates Principles" to condition the entire body, and provide proper alignment, centering, concentration, control, precision, breathing and flowing movement. Pilates has become popular because it is safe; it addresses the foundation of all physical activity, and it is universal in its application to athletics or the work environment.

Proper alignment is essential for strength, efficiency of movement, and prevention of injury. Centering is a concept that states that your core forms the base for all physical movements and that peripheral strength and energy begins at the center of your body. Concentration is important to ensure that movements are performed with precision and control. The principle of controlled breathing reinforces the role of the respiratory and circulatory systems to deliver oxygen and remove waste. Once mastered, these principles should flow together.

Curves is a health and fitness program that was created specifically for women. It has more than 4 million members and widespread appeal. It offers a complete fitness and nutritional system. It works multiple muscle groups and combines cardiovascular activity into an efficient 30 minute routine. It improves health and provides both strength and aerobic conditioning benefits.

At Curves, a unique hydraulic system allows strength training that is safe and effective. It provides controlled resistance based on the amount of force given by the individual. In this way, it safely improves strength.

If less force is applied at a particular point in the range of motion due to weakness or injury then less resistance is given back by the machine. Combine this with their common sense approach to weight management, and their clients greatly improve their fitness level.

Core strengthening is a concept that has been around for more than 80 years. Recently, however, the importance of recognizing the core muscles as the "powerhouse" of your body has gained more attention. The core muscles form the base of support for all that we do. Fine peripheral movements as well as static and dynamic balance all originate from our core.

Your core muscles are the central muscles of your abdomen, pelvis and back. Many exercise programs exist to target your core. In general, you must target all of the muscles at the base of your spine with a circumferential approach. This includes your pelvic floor muscles, abdominal muscles and spine extensors as well as secondary core muscles such as your gluteal muscles, upper back and side muscles. Just like when you are doing arm and chest strengthening, it is easy to neglect the muscles that you don't see reflected back in your mirror.

Postural training is a philosophy practiced by physicians and therapists to correct a flexed posture that is common with a sedentary lifestyle. An evaluation done by a clinician will help to clarify what muscles are weak or inflexible and devise a program of postural training to correct these deficiencies. Often the initial presentation to a physician is a patient with back pain and a flexed, rounded shoulder posture. Back pain will decrease when posture is improved and forces are transmitted in a more ideal manner.

Posture is the position you are in when you are still as well as when you perform movements. These movements may be as basic as sitting at a desk typing or walking down the street. Our posture has important effects on the stresses that are placed on our body. These stresses may lead to anything from low back pain to tension headaches. Stretch and strengthen your muscles to prevent muscle tightness and weakness. These imbalances lead to poor posture, more muscle tightness and weakness, and result in pain and decreased performance.

Spine stabilization is important to prevent injury in both the short and long term. Kirkaldy-Willis established an elegant concept of the degenerative cascade. This degeneration occurs in your spine over many years. With instability of the spine, inappropriate forces are placed on supporting structures. The body responds by trying to stabilize the spine. It does so in an imperfect manner by forming bony osteophytes or calcifying supporting ligaments. This leads to pain and dysfunction.

Much of this degenerative cascade can be slowed if the spine is balanced and supported. The way in which it is supported is analogous to the structure of a tent. The central bony spinal column represents the center pole and the surrounding muscles, soft tissues and extremities are the fabric of the support system. They need to have the right amount of strength and tension to adequately support the bony spine.

Spine flexion and extension exercises are both essential to balance your support system. In most cases, either flexion or extension needs to be emphasized. A trained professional can evaluate your unique situation in order to identify specific imbalances. He or she can then prescribe exercises to correct areas of tightness or weakness so you can function at your highest level and avoid pain and injury.

Sciatic pain, or pain that radiates down one of your extremities, is usually best treated by extension exercises. The classic form of these is McKenzie exercises. These exercises decrease the pressure on the anterior part of your spinal canal thereby decreasing the compression forces through the intervertebral discs. These compressive forces cause discs to bulge or herniate and irritate the sciatic nerve. For patients that have developed spinal stenosis or narrowing of the spinal canal, the prescribed exercises are much different. For these patients, flexion exercises are more appropriate as they can help to open the neural foramina or the paths that the spinal nerves pass through.

Balance, both static, and dynamic, is a critical component of any exercise philosophy. Static balance is the ability to respond to external forces and maintain your equilibrium. Dynamic balance utilizes forces while in motion to keep you upright. Proprioception is the sense of the relative position of neighboring parts of your body. You receive constant conscious and unconscious feedback to create your position sense. Proprioceptive training improves your sense of dynamic balance and improves function and performance.

The Biomechanical Ankle Platform System or "Baps Board" is an example of dynamic proprioceptive training. It improves your lower limb and ankle strength and range of motion while you stand on an exercise platform. It provides neuromuscular reeducation through multiple joints which aids injury healing and prevention of future injuries. For rehabilitation, the size of the pivot ball is gradually increased as healing occurs and function improves.

Theraball exercises are a safe, effective therapeutic tool. Core strengthening of your abdominal and back muscles is more effective on the ball than it is on a mat. The added component of controlling the rolling movement of the ball significantly increases the effectiveness of the strengthening exercises. You are forced to contract your core muscles in multiple different planes to maintain control. To do crunches, lay with your back on the ball with your knees bent to 90 degrees and lift your head and chest approximately 30 degrees. To do back extension exercises, lay with stomach on the ball and reverse the motion. To increases the number of muscles being treated simultaneously, add upper extremity dumbbell exercises to your Theraball routine.

Cost and efficiency of exercise routines are two important factors in our busy lives. The Theraball is an inexpensive piece of exercise equipment that can be purchased and used almost anywhere. It is an efficient exercise tool because it strengthens and stretches multiple areas of your body.

Aquatic exercises are another beneficial form of exercise. They provide resistance and endurance exercises in an unweighted environment with little impact across your joints. The social nature of aquatic exercises is an added benefit. Many locations offer adequate exercise programs directed by a swim instructor or by a physical therapist for more individualized care.

Aquatic exercises are a great form of exercise for all people because of the low impact forces. They are ideal, however, for patients that have painful, arthritic joints or for those who have mobility limitations. They allow exercise of a painful extremity through a range of motion that would never be possible on land. These benefits will lead to improved mobility and decreased pain with all daily activities. Arthritis patients can stabilize a weak, arthritic joint by performing water exercises. This in turn decreases their pain and slows the joint's degeneration.

Performance gains and injury prevention signify the long term success of any exercise program. Don't perform exercises that lead to acute or chronic injuries. Perform low-impact aerobics that lead to a sustained elevated heart rate. High impact aerobics are usually not indicated for the average person trying to stay in shape.

The underlying goal of aerobics is sustained heart rate elevation. Elevated heart rate forces your body to consume more oxygen. In so doing, you improve and maintain aerobic condition. Challenge yourself to find an activity that enables you to do this without causing excessive wear and tear on your joints.

Swimming provides strength, postural and aerobic conditioning. Competitive, high level swimmers achieve great lung capacity and have a tremendous ability to use oxygen. The extension of your spine while swimming also provides great postural benefits. It strengthens your spine extensors and this can have carry over to a more upright posture while on land. The water also provides consistent resistance that strengthens muscles.

Swimming is an activity that can be performed throughout your whole life. It provides a coordinated exercise that can improve strength, posture and flexibility. It avoids the wear and tear that constant impact can cause. Because of this you will see older swimmers with better strength, posture and mobility than their more sedentary counterparts.

Traction used to relieve pain and improve function can be applied in a variety of ways. Inversion tables have become popular recently. In an inversion table, you lock your feet and tilt the table backwards to stretch your spine. This results in a positional form of traction using the forces of gravity to decompress your spine. Manual traction is applied by another practitioner's hands to stretch the patient's soft tissues and relieve pain. Mechanical traction is applied by a piece of equipment. A common mechanism uses hydraulic force applied while you are strapped to the apparatus.

Pain relief with spinal traction occurs through a variety of mechanisms. The stretching may relieve the spasms of painful spinal muscles. It further can slightly distract the spine creating more room for the exiting nerve to pass through the neural foramina. The distractive force creates a vacuum effect that draws bulging discs back into their original configuration. These bulging or herniated discs are often what "pinch" nerves and cause sciatica or radicular pain.

In the following chapter, you will learn how to put together all that you have learned to create relaxed, flowing movement.

CHAPTER 18 - INHERENT MOVEMENT

Mechanical deformities result from abnormal movements and postures. Movements that cause these deformities activate pain-causing elements in soft tissue and supporting structures. Inherent movements are disrupted by abnormal movements and postures and this may lead to pain. The simple act of holding still can block your body's ability to release tension and achieve a point of comfort.

Have you ever noticed how utterly pain free floating can be? Your body is allowed to move where it wants to go and it does not experience resistance. Compare this to the feeling you may have at the end of the day when you feel pain at the base of your neck or in your low back. All day long you have resisted the inherent movement of your body and maintained unnatural postures to do your work activity.

Instinctive, effortless movement is the hallmark of the ideamotor theory or automation. Countless involuntary movements occur as the result of subconscious desires. When assisted, these movements can be used to decrease pain. When resisted, increased sympathetic tone can occur and pain will increase.

These involuntary movements may be influenced by suggestion or expectation. Suggestion may come in the form of a teacher who mandates specific postures or behaviors from her students. Expectation may be from a society that defines appropriate behavior in the workplace. Understand the conscious and unconscious forces that come to bear on you throughout the day and it will ease the chronic discomfort you feel. Suggestions that we receive throughout the day as well as the cumulative suggestions we have amassed over our lifetime guide our behavior and movement in ways we may never be aware.

Utilize the inherent movements that our bodies produce to achieve natural pain relief. Barrett Dorko, P.T., who writes about "The Analgesia of Movement", demonstrates how inherent movements, when released, can decrease pain. Society's edict to maintain a still, upright posture is the origin of this pain. We learn as children, often to our detriment, to suppress our body's instinctive and corrective movements.

Injurious effects of suppressing these inherent movements can lead to pain and dysfunction. A common example is the fatigue of neck extensor muscles that can occur when sitting at a desk for hours on end. This can lead to tissue ischemia, muscle spasm and cervicogenic headaches. These are all common symptoms among office workers. Allow your body to move more in the direction of ease throughout the day and it will decrease the pain and discomfort you feel.

Our minds affect movement in countless ways. Most people never think about all the internal and external factors that affect our movement. Consciously, you can improve your comfort level by allowing more freedom of movement. This inherent movement will relax tense tissue, decrease pain and improve function.

The needs of an organized society direct the inhibitions of specific movements. In the workplace or classroom, standards of conduct exist. In some instances, this can be beneficial to maintain order. At the individual level, they may have beneficial long term effects like improving posture. These standards run the risk of becoming detrimental to your health if they cause pain or create a need to consciously suppress a movement that really might not be doing any harm. A harmless example of this would be to allow a fidgeting boy to get up out of his desk for a couple minutes. This movement could improve his attention and focus.

Abnormal movement exists at the core of chronic pain. These movements may be more focal initially but frequently they become widespread. Pain results in muscle guarding which leads to abnormal movement patterns. These patterns may extend into other parts of the body and cause pain, stiffness and weakness in multiple locations. These patterns often persist long after the initial pain-causing event is terminated. Unwinding these abnormal movement patterns needs to occur in order to restore the ability to have balanced, ideamotor movements.

Chronic pain can extend beyond abnormal movement patterns to all aspects of the chronic pain patient's life. Unfortunately the core or essence of the individual with the chronic pain can become the pain itself. Every role that he has throughout the day is affected by his pain. The pain can become the predominant part of each role and overwhelm the role itself. To begin to resolve this complex problem we must restore normal movement both focally and globally.

Anger and inability to forgive are other factors that prevent natural movement and may lead to pain. An inability to let go of hurt feelings or anger will negatively affect your health. The toll on your health when you withhold forgiveness can be high. Higher rates of chronic pain, cancer, heart disease and depression are present in people who cannot forgive.

Forgiveness frees you of the physical and emotional weight that anger and resentment bring. Amish people speak of "letting go" and forgiving the individual. This does not imply that the misdeed is simply excused. At the heart of this is an ability to separate the act from the person. This expression of compassion can be liberating and will lead to a healthier life. Lift the weight of an unhealthy grudge and release unconscious tensions to promote more healthy movement and decrease pain.

Stress can also lead to abnormal movement, create tension and restrict normal motion. Stress creates an environment of increased sympathetic tone. When you are constantly in a fight-or-flight mode, abnormal motion and pain can occur. Faced with an unconscious desire to either fight or run in an environment where you can do neither is a recipe for unhealthiness. At times, these feelings are healthy as they help us to work hard or be up for a task. When we are unable to turn them off, they become pathological and may lead to abnormal motion, fatigue, and pain.

Stress affects people differently and may settle in different parts of your body. Health professionals should partner with you to try to figure out the ways in which stress has caused abnormal motion or dysfunction of a specific region of your body. You can then work to restore normal movement to that region and counteract the stress effects on that structure.

Relaxation is the first step needed to release abnormal motion. To begin, consciously direct relaxing energy to the body part you want to relax. Concentrate on a particular area and let relaxation occur. To assist this process, practice breathing exercises to train your diaphragm and chest muscles to work more efficiently. The beneficial effects of deep respiration can improve relaxation throughout the body. Add progressive muscle relaxation to further aid this process. To perform this technique, slowly contract and then relax your major muscle groups individually. Pause to pay attention to painful areas.

Visualization is another way to improve relaxation. As a means of self-hypnosis, you can visualize the goal you wish to achieve. This may be pain-free movement, deep sleep or even a high level of performance in a work or athletic endeavor. You need to first achieve an ability to consciously release the tension that is impeding normal movement and function. Following this, begin to visualize success.

Symmetry and balance are important components of movement. Symmetry refers to an equal side to side distribution of body parts. It refers to size, strength and many other factors. In the body, symmetry is approximate as your two halves rarely match up exactly. For efficiency of movement, however, it is a reasonable goal to try to come as close to this as possible. Decreased performance and injury can occur when there is too great of a discrepancy between strength and motion from one side to another.

To achieve balance, assess any side to side differences. Asymmetrical strength differences may occur with long term use of equipment that allows you to significantly favor one extremity when doing the exercise. It is also possible for significant range of motion deficits to occur if one side is tighter than the other or if rotational abnormalities exist.

Oxygenation of tissues occurs through a complex mechanism beginning with the breath we take and continues through the delivery of oxygenated blood by the artery. Although breathing is usually an unconscious, inherent action, abnormal respiration can negatively impact your health. To improve oxygen exchange and have more flowing, relaxed respiration, focus on your respiratory diaphragm. The diaphragm is a large muscle that extends across your rib cage at the base of your chest. To perform abdominal breathing, expand your abdomen during inhalation to move the diaphragm inferiorly. Learn to do abdominal breathing because it creates negative pressure, increases the volume of the chest and draws in more oxygen.

Improved respiration allows more efficient delivery of oxygen and removal of carbon dioxide. It assists removal of waste by the venous and lymphatic structures. The lymphatic vessels that follow the air passages as well as those that run in the soft tissue or connective tissue can better do their job if there is ideal respiratory movement. Learn breathing exercises and you will receive many beneficial effects on your health.

The way in which you move your body, or "body mechanics," is important to improve function and prevent injury. When lifting, distribute the load correctly to decrease the stress that is put upon your body. Lift an object held close to your body to greatly reduce the amount of force that is transmitted to your spine. When at rest, maintain a posture that decreases the amount of force transmitted through your spine. Good posture means your spine is in a neutral position and natural curves are maintained. Over time, abnormal body mechanics can permanently alter the structural integrity of the spine and lead to abnormal motion and pain.

Body mechanics also applies to our extremities. You frequently hear even professional athletes talk about mechanical problems that affect their performance and cause pain. A pitcher, for example, will study hours of video in order to detect a subtle flaw in their mechanics which may have adversely affected their performance or led to pain. It may involve motion that results in inefficient use of the muscles and supporting structures needed to perform the action. Ultimately the goal is to perform at the highest level with the least amount of stress on your body.

Learn to listen to your body because it is important for long term health. Do not deny the subtle signals that your body is sending you and learn to distinguish the clues that you are feeling. Take time to change positions when sitting while doing work in order to avoid the back and neck pain and fatigue that can result from holding a prolonged sitting posture Move in a natural but coordinated manner throughout the day. Allow your instinctive, ideamotor and creative movements that your body needs to release stress. When exercising, try to learn the difference between good and bad pain. A dull muscle ache that results from muscle strength training usually means that you are building muscle. A sharp pain in muscles or joint pain may mean you need to alter your routine.

As noted earlier, small children can teach us a great deal about movement. Unencumbered by social restrictions they allow their bodies to move in a natural way. If you watch them dance or play they tend to move in the way they feel. They will move in the direction they are pulled until an adult "corrects" them. A child tends to move when he or she wants to and not coincidently they have much less pain. As an infant, they learn about their environment by moving, seeing and touching all that is around them. They do not comprehend that the outside world may care how they move so they act how they feel.

As you grow and mature you learn in the context of your environment how you are supposed to act. Unfortunately many of the constraints that are placed upon you lead to unhealthy behaviors and movement patterns. A whole subspecialty of medical science called ergonomics has arisen designed to optimize human well-being and system performance within your environment. At its core are natural, balanced movements and postures within the work environment. This is a worthy goal for any environment in which we live.

In the concluding chapter, I will summarize what we've covered and give you a blueprint for health and fitness.

SUMMARY

Take care of yourself along the journey of your life to achieve your ultimate goal of good health. In 1948, the World Health Organization defined health as a state of complete physical, mental and social well-being and not merely the absence of disease or infirmity. Illness is a state of distress. Health goes beyond the absence of distress or dysfunction to a state of optimum function and well being.

Your ultimate goal should be to take good care of yourself. This truth lies at the center of the definition of health. Good health influences multiple facets of your life and can improve your physical, mental and social well-being. Exercise is a key component of good health. It allows us to fulfill the many roles we assume throughout the day. When examined and applied correctly, it can lead to greater individual satisfaction and improved lifestyle of communities at large.

Distress is a subjective, personal experience that can only by completely understood by the individual. Illnesses, as well as pain, are difficult to quantify. Multiple factors, including physical, emotional, psychological, mental and intellectual well-being and functioning, are diminished or impaired in a state of illness. Illness at times can be felt to be a betrayal by our bodies and as such it affects our trust in ourselves.

Achieve a state of health and minimize disease and you will find that it is a transformative process. For many, it can result in a complete change in identity. Combine all the aspects of health ideally and it will result in a state in which you focus minimal energy on ailments. You are freed to fulfill the other roles in your life without the negative intrusions of pain or sickness.

Perceptions of suffering greatly affect the manner in which suffering is experienced. Whether or not you perceive it as useful determines how much it affects your well-being. Suffering through arduous workouts when you can clearly see a goal at the end of the tunnel is completely different than chronic, useless suffering that is perceived as inevitable. Chronic suffering may result in a defeated attitude which makes it all the more difficult for the suffering to end. In these situations, you need to accept a degree of suffering and minimize the significance of the suffering. The goal of pain management is to reinterpret suffering and place it in a different, less significant context.

For many patients suffering from chronic pain, their suffering begins to assume a larger and larger part of their identity. Envision the roles in your life as overlapping circles. As the circle of pain grows larger, the adjacent areas are compressed. With time, these more important roles may lose their significance.

Rehabilitation medicine can maximize health for all people. A rehabilitation treatment plan begins by identifying individual impairments, the disabilities they cause, and ultimately the handicap which may result. Our goal as Physical Medicine Physicians is to maximize personal function despite illness or injury.

An impairment is any loss or abnormality of a structure or function. Examples include things you can see or touch like a loss of a limb or a sensory deficit. Disability is defined as the loss of ability to perform a specific task because of the impairment. Handicap results through the interaction of the person with the disability in their environment.

Rehabilitation professionals address the individual at all of these different levels. We do what we can to diminish impairments acutely and to maximize healing. To minimize the degree of disability, we work on adaptations or therapies to enable the individual to better perform specific tasks or activities. We address handicap with a global perspective and a willingness to consider everything that affects the ability to fulfill our role in society. Factors include physical, psychosocial and architectural barriers that increase the disadvantage for the individual.

Rehabilitation professionals coordinate their efforts to help a patient achieve their goals. We work within a multidisciplinary or interdisciplinary team model. In the interdisciplinary model, multiple professionals, including doctors and therapists bring their individual talents and goals and mold them in a synergistic manner into a unified plan of care. By working in a coordinated manner, the sum of each individual's contribution is more than each part.

Measurable goals are set by the rehabilitation team and progress is measured. These may be specific mobility goals or they may be higher level functioning goals. The team meets regularly to grade its progress. Specific barriers to achieve these goals are discussed by the team and a plan of care is devised. Methods to achieve these goals may include focused strengthening exercises, adaptive equipment, home modification or family training. The rehabilitation physician coordinates the steps needed to reach the goals.

The initial step of the rehabilitation process should be an evaluation by a rehabilitation physician. This consists of a history and physical examination followed by any appropriate testing, such as x-rays. This evaluation forms the basis of our plan of care and directs treatment. It may focus on a specific part of the body or whole organ system, like the cardiopulmonary system. Therapeutic exercise is the hallmark of treatment. We use exercise to treat an ailment just like we would prescribe a medicine. It may be needed to strengthen a muscle or improve range of motion or endurance. The goal is to have you resume normal tasks and roles with or without modification.

Modify your physical, psychological and social environment to prevent disability. Therapeutic exercise is helpful but it has to be understood within the context of the environment in which you live. Optimal physical strength, psychological balance and environmental accessibility decrease the effect of your impairment. Imbalance in one area can seriously impede function of the other.

We assess the degree of disability by measurements of function. An honest assessment is done in order to measure the functional level, assign a prognosis and set goals. The level of function is affected by multiple internal and external factors. After measuring initial function, we can chart a course to minimize the effects of the functional impairments.

Adaptive equipment consists of many devices such as bedside commodes, walkers, tub benches, or reachers. These allow people with disabilities to often function at a modified independent level. At this level, they can complete the task by themselves when using a device. Sometimes home modifications such as ramps or railings need to be made to remove barriers to function within the home. Family training is needed as well to teach caregivers to provide the appropriate amount of assistance to give to maximize the patient's independence.

ADL's, activities of daily living, or self-care tasks are the essential tasks that we all must perform each day. It is a universal goal in our society to complete these tasks as independently as possible. Eating is an essential ADL. People value the ability to feed themselves so rehabilitative exercises and adaptive equipment are directed towards this goal. Dressing for a disabled person may require adaptive equipment or caregiver assistance. Bathing is another example of an ADL that can be taken for granted by an able-bodied person.

The goals of the individual are paramount for all of these ADL's Cultural bias and unique values affect the practices and habits practiced. Although they may be approached from different points of view, virtually everyone wants to attain the highest level of independence with regards to ADL's following an injury or debilitating illness.

A vocation is defined as your life's work. It is a unique environment or occupation for which an individual is suited or qualified. For some people, it is more than a job but rather something they have been called to do. Vocational rehabilitation recognizes this. It plays an essential role in returning the individual back to the work environment if at all possible. As is done with many other aspects of rehabilitation, goals are evaluated and a plan is put in place to reach them. Barriers to employment need to be overcome.

Transitional work environments exist which allow people to slowly re-enter the work environment. To be successful, appropriate restrictions need to be written by the physician. These may be physical restrictions such as no lifting over 20 pounds or cognitive restrictions such as task simplification. Over time, the goal is for the worker to transition back to full duty. In general, it is best to return an injured worker earlier back to a modified work environment than stay home completely off work.

Psychosocial functioning and well-being greatly affects an individual's disability. All of the rehabilitation team members must tune in to the psychosocial aspects of the rehabilitation plan. The patient's psychosocial functioning includes mood, coping and family interactions. The ultimate goal is to maximize the patient's ability to fulfill all of their roles.

Adjustment to disability counseling is an important part of the rehabilitation process. Adjustment refers to the disabled individual's satisfaction with or acceptance of this circumstance. The disability may result in a loss of work or social status. Change what can be changed and accept what cannot in order to effectively adjust to disability. The most successful disabled individuals constantly confront and overcome obstacles. They assume new roles and figure out adjustments needed to realize their optimum potential.

People need to be willing able to adapt to successfully co-exist in their environment. This is a constant, ongoing process which usually occurs in incremental steps. At times, such as a major trauma or severe injury, the need to adapt quickly occurs. To adapt, either the individual or the environment needs to change. We adapt by doing exercises to become stronger or use adaptive equipment. We change our environment by installing ramps or changing structures to accommodate our needs.

A disability changes our relationship with our environment in a profound way. We are suddenly faced with a new body in the same environment. Environments provide the settings for human activities ranging from large scale group activities down to an individual's life. To interact successfully in our environment, we make modifications that minimize the overall effect of our disability and decrease our handicap.

"Above all, do no harm" is a quote taken from the Hippocratic Oath. Rehabilitation professionals must always keep this in mind. Actions are taken deliberately for the good of the patient. Many alternative treatments must be looked at with a critical eye. This includes supplements such as herbs or vitamins. Some of them can be beneficial but some contain ingredients which could do harm.

We enable the individual to be an active participant in their care to ensure a better outcome and avoid harm. We create a partnership, through education about diet, exercise or environmental modifications to enable the individual to make choices that improve his life. This begins with first doing no harm and progresses ideally to a point where you can realize your full potential.

A biopsychosocial model examines biological, psychological and social aspects of functioning. It entails thoughts, emotions and the ability to fulfill roles. It is in contrast to a biomedical model that suggests that disease processes should be explained simply in terms of an injury, pathogen or some genetic or developmental abnormality. The biopsychosocial model better fits the rehabilitation concept. It is an approach that considers the three important aspects of function and the effects they have on the individual.

Optimize biological aspects of disability to maximize function. Treat disease processes or musculoskeletal conditions first. Ignore the mind-body or psychosocial effects; however, and you ignore a significant factor in health. Once the body and mind have been addressed, evaluate the social ramifications of the condition. We approach a rehab goal from all three perspectives to increase the chance for success.

Cellular injury occurs at a microscopic level due to trauma unleashing a myriad of responses that are as complex as they are unpredictable. As rehabilitation professionals, we are more interested in the disability that results from the impairment than we are the specific injury. We treat the symptoms, minimize the degree of handicap and help to enable our patients to realize their full potential.

The desire to realize your full potential applies to elite and casual athletes as well as people with disabilities. Careful analysis uncovers the most disabling factors. For some people, this may result in marked improvements in sports-specific performance. For a disabled person, it may be the difference between living independently versus in a care center. The analysis is comprehensive in nature and ranges from specific anatomic modifications such as a shoe lift for a leg length discrepancy to architectural changes such as a wheelchair ramp.

Exercise is the key to all you need to do to stay healthy. Because of all the conveniences in our modern society, you must incorporate exercise into your life. Generations past stayed fit simply by doing all they needed to do throughout their day. They would walk to work, perform manual labor, gather and prepare food. In order to stay healthy in today's world, you must make a point of scheduling exercise, stretching and sensible eating into your days.

In summary, you are the only one who decides how you move through life. The thousands of choices that you make all add up to determine how healthy you will be and what quality of life you have. It is not about dieting this month or making a resolution to begin exercising when it warms up. It's about the choices that you make right now. Choose the right thing. Stay fit and achieve your full potential.

At age 15, my life changed drastically. I was thrust into the world of rehabilitation in a way that I could have never imagined.

EPILOGUE

Graduating from medical school and beginning a residency in Physical Medicine and Rehabilitation was the pinnacle of a journey that began at the lowest point in my life. At age 15, I suffered a cervical spinal cord injury known as a Brown-Séquard injury. It left me unable to walk and barely able to move my left arm. It was the beginning of a road of discovery for me that would make me more determined than ever to excel.

Two years after my injury, this road led me to college to study pre-medicine with a new-found interest in the medical field. After college, I completed a thesis in graduate school entitled "Low-Back Strength Testing and the Probability of Low-Back Pain Management". At that point, I still didn't consciously realize how my earlier experience had led me down that path. Following Graduate School, I entered Osteopathic Medical School. After this, I began a residency in Physical Medicine and Rehabilitation and ultimately become a practicing Physiatrist.

How the injury happened remains a mystery. It was early in a regular day of wrestling practice and we were doing routine mat drills. I felt a strange numbness and weakness and I told my coach that I was having trouble moving and feeling my hands. When I went to stand up, I realized that I couldn't. My legs felt like they were not there and I had to be helped to the trainers room.

My weakness progressed rapidly at that point. Whether my spinal cord had been bruised or stretched, a cascade had been unleashed and every part of my body below my neck was being affected. What began as something that we thought could be treated with Icy Hot being rubbed on my stiff hands quickly became an emergency.

The first ambulance that responded did not recognize the severity of the situation. One of the paramedics felt that he needed to repeatedly check a Babinski reflex by scratching the sole of my foot with a safety pin. Although I did not feel it, he left me with multiple linear abrasions on the sole of my foot. Their slow and callous manner taught me first-hand how vulnerable a patient can feel.

What began as a normal day in my sophomore year in high school ended with me being transported by a second ambulance to the hospital. I was transformed in an instant from someone who played three sports my previous year in high school to being someone who could barely move. It was a surreal scene as I looked up into the eyes of my concerned and curious classmates as I was being carried out of the school on a stretcher.

That night began a grueling journey on the road to recovery. In 1981, CT scans and MRI's were not available so I underwent a myelogram. After enduring the painful procedure, I found myself too weak to lift my head to throw up from the nausea the dye had caused. The diagnosis of a cervical spinal cord injury was eventually made primarily by a history and physical exam.

After my injury, I spent one month in the children's hospital. I learned first hand the profound effect caring therapists can have. They worked with me every day to help me regain my strength and I made rapid improvements. After a few weeks, still unable to walk, I was devastated to learn that I would be going home in a wheelchair. After some pleading, the doctors agreed to let me stay another week. I redoubled my efforts and was ultimately discharged home walking with a quad cane.

After my accident, therapy became a regular part of my life for the next 18 months. My initial status was strict bed rest but it progressed quickly to intensive inpatient rehabilitation. After discharge from the hospital, I worked with an exercise physiologist for a year and a half. This was the same group of people who would eventually provide me with much of the data I needed to write my Masters Thesis seven years later. Call it good karma.

When I walked for the first time in nearly four weeks, it was a strange and wonderful experience. I walked initially with the aid of a walker. I was struck by the fact that I had to think about what had been automatic since I was one year old. I continued to strengthen my muscles over the following year with Cybex weight machines. I learned that I could compensate for muscles that had permanently lost their nerve supply and strengthen other areas.

My Return home from the hospital unleashed a series of emotions in me as I realized that life as I knew it and the image of myself had profoundly changed. Being re-introduced to people I hadn't seen for over a month was strange in so many ways. My toddler cousin ran towards me when I was sitting on the floor and knocked me over as if we were the same size. I had been so strong. I was used to taking down other wrestlers and now I was taken down by someone weighing no more than 25 lbs.

The low point came for me when I was doing exercises with my mom the week I returned home from the hospital. I was feeling so strongly the loss I had experienced that I just started to cry. Fortunately for me, she looked back at me with all the strength and love in the world and just said, "Come on. Let's get to work." I promised myself that day to never feel sorry for myself again.

My sense of loss first hit me like a ton of bricks when I went home. I sensed these impending feelings when they mentioned discharge home the first time from the hospital. I didn't want to go home and I pleaded for them to let me stay. In the hospital, I was shielded from reality. Although it was inevitable, I didn't want to be confronted with all of the things that I could no longer do. One of the most painful losses that sill bothers me to this day was my loss of the ability to play my guitar. I was no Jimi Hendrix but I had enjoyed playing for many years in a contemporary mass group and I thought it was something I would do my whole life With the loss of strength and coordination in my left hand, playing was difficult and I never achieved my previous skill.

I realized I had lost much of my speed and strength when I returned home from the hospital. When I returned home, I was walking with a quad cane. As I progressed to running, it was clear how much slower I had become. Growing up, I had always had good strength and fitness. In grade school, I had earned the Presidential Physical Fitness Award every year I was eligible even though I rarely received an individual award for being the best in a single event. To the average person who had not known me prior to my injury, they may suspect little but going forward, every thing I did physically had changed.

Body image for a teenager under even the best of circumstances can at times be a dicey proposition. With all the changes an adolescent goes through, it is easy to be overly se-conscious and critical of the image you see looking back at you in the mirror. For me, the dramatic change in the shape of my body was impossible to avoid. The loss of my chest or pectoral muscles seemed particularly dramatic. I watched them melt away before my eyes when I was in the hospital. Coupled with this was the fact that my muscle loss was asymmetrical, effecting my left side to a much larger degree than my right.

When I returned to the soccer fields the following year, I made a huge step on the path to returning to my normal life. Although my ability to play at a high level was gone, I was still able to get out onto the field and participate. Throughout the year, I arrived late to practice because I was attending exercise physiology at the hospital after school. I went three days a week to therapy to try to regain some of my strength. Afterwards, I would just show up late and try to slip into the practice routine. The support given to me by my high school coaches was phenomenal.

The following year, I was elected junior varsity co-captain as a testament to my hard work and determination, more so than my on the field performance. Because my injury primarily affected my left side, I was able to compensate and use mainly my right leg when I played. My hard work coupled with this fact provided me some degree of effectiveness. Unfortunately it resulted in my right leg becoming even more disproportionately stronger than my left leg .One day when I was bending it into the net on corner kicks, one of the freshmen said to me "Man you would have really been something if that hadn't happened to you". In a bittersweet way, that made me feel good

As I grew older I compensated for the strength differences by only working my right side as hard as my left when doing weight lifting activities because I didn't want to amplify my right sided strength advantage. If I'm doing curls, I use the same weight and do the same number of reps side to side. I stress the importance of this principle with my patients as well. Frequently you need to target a week area with exercise and don't let a stronger area overcompensate. There are both functional and cosmetic reasons to exercise this way as the weaker area will be more susceptible to injury.

During the 15 years following my injury, I exercised inconsistently. I played a variety of recreational sports, lifted eights casually and jogged periodically. I found myself incredibly busy with school, and then work and exercise fell lower on my list in terms of importance. I didn't have any particular fitness goals at that time in my life and I had never had a weight problem so it wasn't a big issue to me. Because of my altered biomechanics, I suffered a stress fracture in my left foot playing basketball which caused pain and slowed me down for a while. With the spasticity that developed on my left side, I tend to come down more on the ball of my left foot which places abnormal stress across the bones of my foot which led to my fracture.

It is easy to see how if you don't commit to exercise, it can easily be neglected. You really need to "pay yourself first "and make exercise a priority. For a busy person, exercise needs to be scheduled. The importance of exercise as you grow older cannot be overemphasized because it affects all aspects of your life. It enables you to stay healthier and fulfill al of your roles more successfully.

In my late thirties, I made a commitment to exercise regularly. My decision was influenced by completing a residency in Physical Medicine and Rehabilitation. It became hard to ignore in my own life the messages I was giving to my patients. I also experienced a rekindled desire to compete. Although I had never been much of a long-distance runner, my brother invited me to run a 5K with him one New Years eve. I enjoyed the competition both against others as well as the clock more than I had expected. After that, I became a regular participant in a couple races a year. I realized that I was never going to be one to win any more races but I knew I could be competitive and running offered me an opportunity to exercise and compete with no particular time constraints.

With a new found realization that I could compete, consistent physical activity became my goal. I rarely do the same thing for an extended period of time. If I become extremely busy with everything else in my life, I'll try to sneak in brief workouts in my basement or do quick floor exercises before work. I'll also mix more activity into my daily routine by doing things like parking further away or taking the steps instead of the elevator. To remain flexible, I slip brief stretches into periods of down time. These activities combine to avoid the rollercoaster of weight and conditioning changes. Variety mixed with consistency also helps to avoid overuse injuries as well as the boredom that may come with repeating the same routine.

When investing money, financial advisors tell you that no matter what you must always pay yourself first. This same philosophy applies when you are on an airplane and the stewardess tells you to place the oxygen mask on yourself first and then the child. You must take care of yourself in order to be able to serve others. You must make caring for yourself a priority. Consistent exercise through good times and bad is synonymous with dollar cost averaging. The benefits will grow and accumulate and dividends will be paid over the long run even though there will inevitably be down times.

It is tempting to want to postpone exercise to a point in your life when you feel you may have more time. In our busy society, unfortunately, that time may never come. Just like saving for retirement, if you wait until you feel like you have extra money lying around to invest, this may never occur. You must pay yourself the time or money off the top and don't even figure it into the rest of the day. Consider it the cost of doing business. Fortunately with exercise, the possibilities to do this are endless and the time or money invested will provide great returns.

I realized in my 30's that even with my impairments, I could still perform many sports activities at a high level Breaking 23 minutes in a 5K race was a great accomplishment for me. It placed me in the upper quartile for my age group in spite of the fact that I didn't run nearly as many miles on a regular basis a many of the other contestants. Tennis was anther sport in which I could excel because it was primarily a right handed sport and was less likely to expose my weaknesses. Soccer remains a sport that I truly enjoy. I was able to compete because success in soccer depends in large part on your fitness level. The ability to run long distances separates you from other players as you approach middle age.

Because my injury occurred in my sophomore year in high school, I never physically peaked at a young age like so many athletes do. I don't have any great high school athletic glory to remember or satisfy me. Because of that, I've spent my adult life motivated to continue to improve in many different areas. It continuously amazes me how with sports and exercise, you can always find something that will keep you coming back for more. Ask any golfer what a few great shots in a round of golf does to their desire to get back out on the links. You must continue to make small goals for yourself and recognize little victories you may have achieved even when no one else notices.

People diverge in many different ways as they age. Some of this is due to our genetics but much of it is dependant upon our diet and exercise habits. The path we choose is up to us. Insidious weight gain can slowly rob us of much of our mobility and athletic ability. Before you know it, you may be looking down at a large belly wondering where it came from. Maintain an ideal weight both for health and mobility reasons. If you store large amounts of fat, it will affect your physical performance as well as the overall health and function of your internal organs.

Many athletes excel in violent sports at a young age because of their size and strength. Unfortunately, they pay for it years later with chronic pain and decreased mobility. All of the hits they absorbed and the severe stresses that they placed across their joints cause accelerated wear and tear on their bodies. The large size that they achieved no longer serves them well in a more sedentary middle age. To reverse this path, they need to focus on lower weight, toning exercises and aerobic conditioning.

It is interesting to observe people years later that had looked so young and skinny in their teen years. Many of them maintain their youthful appearance by staying thin and active. If you choose the path of lifelong fitness and participate in appropriate activities, it will enable you to live a long and active life. If that is the path you choose, there are few reasons why you can't stay physically active and mobile late into life.

Fate threw me a curve at age 15 that left me feeling devastated and lost. In the months that followed I dealt with the pain and loss by just trying not to feel anything. I pushed forward, denying that things had changed. They had changed for me, however and things could never be the same. As much as I wanted my old life back, I new that things were different. I was buoyed by a great deal of love and support from my teammates, coaches and families at my high school. Although I felt uncomfortable with the standing ovations they gave me at sports banquets, I must admit that I appreciated the fact that they recognized what I had gone through.

Choices we make in life are based on our cumulative knowledge and experiences up until that point. Although I didn't directly relate it at the time, my injury was instrumental in my decision to become a doctor and ultimately go into Rehabilitation Medicine. It just felt natural to me. I feel I can be more sensitive to people with disabilities and relate to some of their unique challenges. I also feel comfortable in challenging them to overcome their disabilities and to be successful at whatever they want to do. I learned to appreciate what an awesome thing is the human body and to not live a day without being grateful for all that it enables us to do, We're only given one, so you better take care of it.

RESOURCES

Books

Anderson, Bob. *Stretching* (updated edition). Bolinas, CA: Shelter Publications, 2000.

Peeke, Pamela. *Fit to Live.* New York, NY: Rodale Books, 2007.

Karas, Jim. *The 7 Day Energy Surge.* New York, NY: Rodale Books, 2009.

Heavin, Gary. *Curves.* New York, NY: Penguin Group (USA), 2003.

Dorko, Barrett L. *The Analgesia of Movement: Ideamotor Activity and Manual Care.* IJOM, Volume.6, Issue 2. Elsevier Inc. Philadelphia, PA: October 2003.

Van Buskirk, Richard L. DO, PhD. *Still Technique Manual,* 2nd edition, American Academy of Osteopathy, Indianapolis, IN 2006.

Ward, RC. *Foundations for Osteopathic Medicine,* Ward, RC (ed) (2003). Williams and Wilkins. Baltimore, MD. 1997.